El Cajon, CA 92019

VOLUME I

INTEGRATIVE
MANUAL THERAPY

FOR THE AUTONOMIC NERVOUS SYSTEM
AND RELATED DISORDERS

Utilizing
Advanced Strain and Counterstrain Technique

Thomas Giammatteo, D.C., P.T.
Sharon Weiselfish-Giammatteo, Ph.D. P.T.

North Atlantic Books
Berkeley, California

Integrative Manual Therapy™
for the Autonomic Nervous System
and Related Disorders

Published by
North Atlantic Books
P.O. Box 12327
Berkeley, California 94712

Cover and book design by Andrea DuFlon

Printed in the United States of America

Integrative Manual Therapy™ *for the Autonomic Nervous System and Related Disorders* is sponsored by the Society for the Study of Native Arts and Sciences, a nonprofit educational corporation whose goals are to develop an educational and crosscultural perspective linking various scientific, social, and artistic fields; to nurture a holistic view of arts, sciences, humanities, and healing; and to publish and distribute literature on the relationship of mind, body, and nature.

3   4   5   6   7   8   9   DATA   10   09   08   07   06

ACKNOWLEDGMENTS

The authors wish to acknowledge Lawrence Jones, D.O., the developer of Strain and Counterstrain Technique, whose research and documentation during half a century contributed an outstanding procedure to health care and the field of manual therapy. Lawrence Jones, Larry to his friends, was a humble and modest man, with integrity and truth as a model for all health care practitioners.

We wish to extend our appreciation to Loren Rex, D.O., who introduced us to Strain and Counterstrain Technique.

We want to extend our gratitude to Carol Gordon, P.T., I.M.P.,C, Jay Kain, Ph.D., P.T., A.T.C., I.M.P.,C, and our colleagues at Regional Physical Therapy in Connecticut, who supported the clinical research in this new area of manual practice to address autonomic nervous system dysfunction.

We extend our respect and appreciation to those original thinkers and developers who influenced us and thereby contributed to the unfolding of this approach: Jean Pierre Barral, D.O., whose research and instruction in visceral manipulation and Listening is a foundation for all our work; Paul Chauffour, D.O., who developed Inhibitory Balance Testing, for more efficient rehabilitation; and Hildegaard Wittlinger, who brought Manual Lymph Drainage to North America.

Many, many thanks to our clients who continue to return for more and improved manual therapy. We will always be here for you.

Thanks and appreciation to John Giammatteo, for your artistry and skill in photography.

Thank you Ayelet Weiselfish and Genevive Pennell, for the gift of your illustrations.

Love and appreciation to Nim, Ayelet, and Amir, our children, whose blessings and encouragement have been such a gift.

And, once again, thank you Margaret Loomer, whose creativity and skill make books.

With Love,
Sharon and Tom

TABLE OF CONTENTS

FOREWORD

Considering the frequency of asthma, hypertension, hypotension, glaucoma, ulcer disease, and abnormalities of sweating, temperature, cardiac rhythm, respiration, sexual, bowel and bladder function, it is amazing that the autonomic system gets essentially no direct treatment. Rather, those symptoms produced by lack of homeostasis of this system have been attacked with a vengeance but with no correction of the problematic system.

Diabetes Mellitus, multiple sclerosis, Guillain-Barre's syndrome and infraction are often associated with disorders of autonomic function. Our medical response has been reduced to a barrage of pharmacological antidotes: antihypertensives, psychotropic drugs, atropinics, alpha- and beta-adrenergic stimulating and inhibiting agents but in no single case is this treatment directed at the problem, only the symptom. None of this central or peripheral clinical pharmacology addresses the system directly.

The autonomic nervous system is the normally involuntary or unconscious division of the peripheral nervous system. Its efferent stimulation of all smooth muscles from blood vessels, lymphatic vessels, organs and glands as well as the resting muscle tone that allows us to sit up is a function of this autonomic nervous system. The autonomic nervous system has two divisions, the sympathetic and the parasympathetic. The parasympathetic system regulates the functions necessary for long term survival. Everything from salivation and digestion to heart rate, respiratory rate, pancreatic function, liver and gallbladder function, and urine excretion through the kidneys, ureters and bladder, are only a few of the things that fall under autonomic control. The sympathetic system meets all crises; it spares no expense. The parasympathetics pick up after the sympathetics, replenishing, restoring and replacing, preparing for a rainy day. And when the parasympathetics can no longer "keep up" all life becomes a crisis and the overload escalates more and more with less and less provocation.

All cells have sympathetic innervation, including blood vessels which, when hypertonic, decrease distribution of oxygen even to the brain in a crisis. The impact of this is reduced healing, increased hypertension, facilitated segments, changes in endocrine function impacting metabolism, brain function and ultimately all homeostatic mechanisms. But when this system is balanced, cells have their optimal potential to repair and replace themselves for an estimated 120–140 years. We die from lack of homeostasis in this system and are disabled when its harmony is simply out of sync. It affects every fiber of our being—so where is the treatment?

Well, you're holding it in your hands! Dr. Sharon Weiselfish-Giammatteo has, using the basic principles of Lawrence Jones' Strain/counterstrain, developed a mechanical/corrective kinesiology model. This technique brought marked changes in her neurologic patients. Dr. Weiselfish-Giammatteo further observed a synergic pattern of spastic muscles whether the client was a pediatric cerebral palsy, geriatric hemiplegic, chronic pain or other patient. When the mechanical model was applied from proximal to distal, to the muscles which contribute directly to the synergic pattern, spasticity and severe protective muscle spasm are remarkably reduced.

When synchronizers (energetic relexogenic points which control and/or inhibit different body functions) were added to the mechanical and synergistic model and held past the ninety seconds of Jones, a "De-Facilitated Fascial Release™" occurred. The resultant tissue "unwinding" occurs secondary to the elimination and/or decrease of hypotonicity and appears to occur at a cellular level, specifically in the ground substance or matrix of the connective tissue. I have found in my clinic after literally thousands of hours of application that a homeostasis is returned to the autonomic system as a direct and immediate response to this treatment.

The body's ability to heal depends on creating a balanced environment in the tissues. This environment is directly controlled by the autonomic system and its balance. Advanced Strain and Counterstrain of the Autonomic Nervous System provides a direct and ongoing impact on the homeostasis of this system thereby creating the environment in which our bodies do what they do best—HEAL. Without autonomic balance, there can be no health, only various levels of dis-ease. I have never worked with any treatment whether it be surgical, pharmacologic or manual therapy which has such an incredible impact on the individual's body. it doesn't just relieve symptoms, it allows for true recovery of the autonomic system. Its simplicity allows it to be managed by all levels from physicians to manual therapists, to patients themselves in certain instance. The work is profound, the results are profound and, when integrated with other directed manual therapies, can establish a state of ongoing health improvement and potential that is limited only by your patience and belief systems.

This text is a jewel, when incorporated into an informed treatment setting, will change your life as a manual therapy practitioner. Your patients will be the recipients of this simple straightforward work that is elegant in its simplicity and lasting in its effects and reproducibility. I have found no contraindication to the work, and done in the proper context it can do no harm. In twenty years in medicine I have never found such a versatile tool and I'm truly excited that it can now be shared with the rest of the world.

Mary A. Lynch, MS, M.D., P.A.
The Center for Sports Medicine and Rehabilitation
Wichita, Kansas

CHAPTER 1

PRESENT MODELS OF
STRAIN AND COUNTERSTRAIN TECHNIQUE

The History of the Phenomenon of Strain and Counterstrain Technique

Since Lawrence Jones, D.O. started his studies and documentation of Strain and Counterstrain Technique in the early 1990's, the art and science of this approach has progressed to the remarkable techniques presented in this text. When he discovered that precise positions would eliminate pain and disability in persons with similar painful postures, he searched for other typical correlations. He detected Tender Points, which were exquisitely painful on palpation, at the exact same locations in all persons with identical postural deviations. He determined that these postural deviations were because of protective muscle spasm. He discerned that the shortened muscles in spasm were pulling on bony articular surfaces, contributing to joint dysfunction. He appreciated that the precise positions which resulted in improved movement and decreased discomfort also dissipated the pain of the Tender Point.

Thus, Dr. Jones began his search for painful Tender Points in the bodies of all of his patients. When he discovered a new painful point which was present in the same exact location in the typical person, his investigation towards finding the precise position to dissipate the pain of this Tender Point ensued. Later he defined the problem: which muscle in spasm was reflected by which Tender Point. During his quest for information he learned that these precise positions would need to be maintained for exactly ninety (90) seconds. Although Lawrence Jones did not understand the neuroscience underlying this clinical phenomenon, his faith and his vision conquered questions of relevance.

Over fifty years of his investigation of

the phenomenon of Strain and Counterstrain generated a comprehensive approach for the treatment of somatic dysfunction and pain. Approximately one hundred and seventy five (175) Tender Points and their correlating precise positions were documented by Dr. Jones. Elimination of muscle spasm with Dr. Jones' Strain and Counterstrain Technique is a phenomenon. The art of this approach is described in several texts by different authors. The science of this procedure is still under investigation.

The following descriptions of the various models of Strain and Counterstrain Technique are presented in order to facilitate extrapolation of this approach for various patient populations.

Jones' Model (Jones)

Lawrence Jones, D.O. was the original developer of Strain and Counterstrain Technique. He spent over half a century perfecting this approach for the treatment of somatic dysfunction. Dr. Jones discovered that there are extremely tender points on the body, which people present in a similar manner. The Tender Points are exhibited in the same exact locations. Each Tender Point is a reflection of a muscle in spasm, or of a joint and/or suture in a state of compression. His discovery that positional therapy would eliminate the pain of the Tender Point led to his further understanding that holding this position for 90 seconds would result in elongation of the muscle and decompression of the joint and/or suture. Dr. Jones created an approach which changes arthrokinematics and osteokinematics in a remarkable manner. Joint mobility and joint play is usually restored with Strain and Counterstrain Technique. Articular balance, which is the relative normal positions of the articular surfaces of a joint during physiologic motion, is improved. Ranges of motion are always increased dramatically. Utilization of this approach educates the practitioner about the normal elongation capacity of a muscle. While documenting his findings during the initial stages of creation, he did not know that his approach worked on decreasing the hyperactivity of the myotatic reflex arc. He believed; he was guided; he followed with humility and with admiration of the results of his creation. Dr. Jones will be remembered for his contribution of enormous proportion to manual therapy.

Mechanical/Corrective Kinesiology Model (Weiselfish-Giammatteo)

Sharon Weiselfish-Giammatteo, Ph.D., P.T., co-author of this text, began to work with Lawrence Jones' Strain and Counterstrain Technique in 1981. Weiselfish-Giammatteo observed how a 90 seconds technique eliminated a 'locked jaw' secondary to a masseter spasm after surgery for parotid gland tumor excision. She began to teach herself this approach from Dr. Jones' book, and learned that many clients with moderate and severe hypertonicity would not experience pain on palpation of the Tender Point. They presented an atypical response to pressure on that point. She began to develop a 'mechanical' model for treatment of patients with atypical pain perception, such as the neurologic, pediatric, geriatric and chronic pain patient. Her development of this model was based on knowledge of kinesiology and muscle function. For example, the pectoralis minor which originates on the second, third and fourth rib, and inserts on the coracoid process, protracts the shoulder girdle. When the shoulder girdle is protracted, the pectoralis muscle is in protective muscle spasm. There will be a limitation of horizontal abduction. Whenever there is a shoulder girdle protraction, the Strain and Counterstrain

technique for the pectoralis muscle (called the second depressed rib, because Lawrence Jones observed that contraction of the pectoralis minor depresses the second rib) will eliminate the postural dysfunction. The protraction of the shoulder girdle will disappear, even if it is severe and chronic. Weiselfish-Giammatteo developed a postural evaluation of sagittal, coronal and transverse plane posture. When postural deviation and limitations of ranges of motion are assessed, a knowledge of kinesiology will determine which muscles are in spasm. When these muscles are treated with Strain and Counterstrain Technique, there is an elongation of the muscle fiber, increased ranges of motion, and a remarkable improvement in postural symmetry.

This mechanical/kinesiologic model works exceptionally well for the neurologic client. For example, a typical dysfunction in a cerebral vascular accident client is a painful subluxation of the glenohumeral joint, described in the literature as a "subluxed hemiplegic shoulder." Berta Bobath defined this disorder as a latissimus dorsi in a state of hypertonicity within a flaccid shoulder girdle after stroke. The latissimus dorsi is the only depressor of the humeral head. When the Strain and Counterstrain technique is used for the latissimus dorsi there will usually be a total reduction of the subluxation of the humeral head, because the latissimus dorsi muscle fibers will elongate, and they will no longer pull on the humeral head in a caudal direction. This approach will be successful in acute and chronic shoulder subluxation, no matter how severe the presentation. The neurologic client requires that the position be held for three (3) to five (5) minutes, rather than for 90 seconds.

Synergic Pattern Release™ Model (Weiselfish-Giammatteo)

Sharon Weiselfish-Giammatteo, Ph.D., P.T., utilized Dr. Jones' Strain and Counterstrain to treat spasticity in the neurologic client, not only to treat protective muscle spasm in the orthopedic-like client. She realized that the hypertonicity of spasticity was similar in nature and characteristics to the hypertonicity of protective muscle spasm. There is primary dysfunction: hyperactivity of the myotatic reflex arc. This hyperactivity is reduced with Strain and Counterstrain Technique, whether the manifestation is protective muscle spasm or spasticity. These techniques require a holding of the positions for three (3) to five (5) minutes, rather than 90 seconds, for optimal results.

Weiselfish-Giammatteo further observed that the synergic pattern of spastic muscles was similar in presentation for all severely impaired clients, whether pediatric cerebral palsy, geriatric hemiplegic, chronic pain or other. When the Strain and Counterstrain techniques are applied proximal to distal, to the muscles which contribute directly to the synergic pattern, spasticity and severe protective muscle spasm is remarkably reduced. For example, the synergic pattern of the upper extremity is as follows: an elevated shoulder girdle; a protracted shoulder girdle; an adducted shoulder in internal rotation; a flexed elbow; a pronated forearm; a flexed wrist in ulnar deviation; flexed fingers; a flexed and adducted thumb. The Strain and Counterstrain techniques can be applied to eliminate the synergic pattern of presentation in the follow-ing sequence: the supraspinatus; the elevated first rib; the pectoralis minor; the biceps; the wrist flexors; the finger flexors; the first metacarpal technique. The spastic synergic pattern can be reduced, and even eliminated, with this approach.

Inhibitory Balance Testing™ and Mechanical Link Model (Chauffour)

Paul Chauffour, D.O. developed a remarkably efficient approach for treatment of somatic, cranial and visceral dysfunction called Mechanical Link™. He created Inhibitory Balance Testing™,

which discovers the primary dominant lesion which is contributing to all of the other lesions in the body. With this approach, the practitioner can find the one major problem in the spinal column, in the rib cage and sternum, in the cranium, in the extremity joints, and in the visceral system which affects the whole person.

Weiselfish-Giammatteo, Ph.D., P.T. and D'Ambrogio, P.T., adapted Chauffour's Inhibitory Balance Testing™ to Jones' Strain and Counterstrain Technique. The Jones' Tender Points are 'balanced' against each other with Inhibitory Balance Testing™. The whole body can be assessed in this manner. The primary, dominant Tender Point will be evident, which indicates which muscle in spasm is contributing to the protective muscle spasm of most of the other muscles. This muscle can be treated with the specific Strain and Counterstrain technique, which will cause a general decrease in the hypertonicity of all of the other muscles.

Also, Weiselfish-Giammatteo discovered 'Muscle Rhythm™.' Muscle Rhythm™ of the major muscles can be assessed and 'balanced' against each other. In this manner, Inhibitory Balance Testing™ can be utilized for Strain and Counterstrain Technique. The muscle with the dysfunctional Muscle Rhythm™ which is contributing to the dysfunctional Muscle Rhythm™ of the other muscles can be treated with Strain and Counterstrain Technique.

Behavioral Modification for Chronic Pain Model (Weiselfish-Giammatteo)

Treatment of clients with chronic pain syndrome is difficult. These persons believe that life without pain does not exist. In order to affect these belief systems, they require proof that pain can be eliminated, and will not return. Behavioral modification can be utilized with Strain and Counterstrain Technique. The practitioner can isolate the Jones' Tender Point. The client can press on the Tender Point and experience the exquisite pain on palpation of the point. The Strain and Counterstrain technique is then performed by the therapist. The patient once again presses on the Tender Point, and finds that there is no longer any pain present. After several repetitions, the client begins to question whether or not pain is a requirement for living!

CHAPTER 2

ALTERNATIVE METHODS
Strain and Counterstrain Technique Combined with Other Approaches

This chapter presents alternate methods for utilization of Strain and Counterstrain Technique. Many unique approaches were developed which can be adapted to use with Jones' procedures.

Inhibitory Balance Testing™ Adapted for Strain and Counterstrain Technique

Strain and Counterstrain Technique is an approach to treat hypertonicity, developed by Lawrence Jones, D.O. Inhibitory Balance Testing™ is an evaluation process to discover dominant restrictions in the body, developed by Paul Chauffour, D.O. Inhibitory Balance Testing™ is an integral component of Mechanical Link™, a manual therapy approach which addresses total body somatic dysfunction. When Inhibitory Balance Testing™ is incorporated into Strain and Counterstrain Technique, the practitioner can determine which muscle, in a state of hypertonicity, is contributing to hypertonicity of other muscles.

It is possible to perform Inhibitory Balance Testing™ in a *regional format* and in a *total body format* utilizing Muscle Rhythm Therapy™ (for explanation of assessment and treatment of Muscle Rhythm™, refer to Chapter 26 of this text: Muscle Rhythm Therapy™). In a *regional format,* the Muscle Rhythm™ of different muscles in a body region, for example, the biceps and triceps of the right upper extremity may be compared. A *nullification process* can determine which muscle is the dominant muscle of that body region. To determine the dominant muscle of the right upper extremity, you palpate the Muscle Rhythm™ of one muscle, the biceps, and then place hand contact on another muscle, the triceps. If the Muscle Rhythm™ of the biceps im-

proves when hand contact is placed on the triceps, the triceps is the dominant muscle. The hypothetical model is such: by placing contact on the triceps, you are inhibiting its negative effect on the biceps and thereby, improving the biceps' function. All muscles in the body can be compared via this method utilizing Muscle Rhythm Therapy™.

When Inhibitory Balance Testing™ is used with the *total body format,* the dominant muscle is determined for each of the following body parts: 1. right lower extremity, 2. left lower extremity, 3. right upper extremity, 4. left upper extremity, 5. abdomen, 6. pelvis and low back, 7. sternum and anterolateral rib cage, 8. upper back, 9. neck, 10. cranium, 11. face.

A nullification process with Inhibitory Balance Testing™ determines, by comparison, which is the primary dominant muscle of the 11 dominant muscle regions remaining, as outlined in the above paragraph. When the muscles which are dominant are treated with Strain and Counterstrain Technique™, the result can be a total elimination of the primary self-perpetuating protective muscle spasm and hypertonicity which is affecting many muscles as well as correction of the Muscle Rhythm™ of all the muscles treated.

Neurofascial Process™ Utilized with Strain and Counterstrain Technique

Neurofascial Process™, developed by Sharon Weiselfish-Giammatteo, Ph.D., P.T., is a differential diagnosis and treatment approach which addresses body and mind dysfunction. This approach allows the practitioner two premises. One premise gives the ability to recognize areas of dysfunction which contribute to the dysfunctions of other parts of the body. Another premise of this work gives the ability to deter-

---

The Process Center for hypertonicity is the mental body (Weiselfish-Giammatteo). The mental body access is approximately 1 cm anterior to/above the left frontal eminence.

---

mine the non-physical process which is part of the physical dysfunction. Certain typical body areas surface as part of the client's problem when emotions, cognitive thoughts, and/or spiritual disturbances are contributing to the symptomatology. These body areas are called *Process Centers*, and present in typical manifestations for similar situations in all persons. The body responds in these Neurofascial Process™ patterns, in a similar behavioral model, for all persons, no matter the age, gender, personal traits.

Strain and Counterstrain Technique with Neurofascial Process™ for Treatment of Hypertonicity

When performing Jones' Strain and Counterstrain Technique, or Advanced Strain and Counterstrain Technique, whatever the etiology (protective muscle spasm, spasticity, other), contact on the *mental body* will augment the outcome. Position the body in the Strain and Counterstrain Technique position (Jones' positions, and also the Advanced Strain/Counterstrain positions by Weiselfish-Giammatteo and Giammatteo). There is an apparent association between the *mental body* energy and the actin/myosin interface of the sarcomere.

When performing Strain and Counterstrain Technique with Neurofascial Process™, hand contact must be maintained on the muscle. The Jones, or Weiselfish-Giammatteo/Giammatteo Strain/Counterstrain position is maintained throughout the technique. Hand contact is maintained at the access of the *mental body*. The

client's hand can maintain this contact, or the hand of another person can be used. After the 90 seconds (1 minute for the Advanced Strain/Counterstrain techniques) there will be continued unwinding of the fascial tissue. Maintain the position and the hand contacts for the duration of the De-Facilitated Fascial Release™.

Synchronizers™ Utilized with Strain and Counterstrain Technique

During her clinical research with manual therapy, Sharon Weiselfish-Giammatteo discovered Synchronizers™ to affect the tissues of the brain and heart. Her work is ongoing, and has culminated in a series of manual therapy courses called Biologic Analogs™, which are presented by Therapeutic Horizons™, a continuing education institution for advanced learning for manual practitioners. Weiselfish-Giammatteo has discovered many Synchronizers™ which facilitate restoration of multiple body functions.

A Synchronizer™ is an energetic reflexogenic point which controls and/or inhibits different body functions. These points are found on the lungs, on the cranium, in the abdomen and low back, and in the pelvic region.

When protective muscle spasm and/or spasticity is diffuse throughout the body, further inhibition of the hyperactive myotatic reflex arc is attained with contact on two (2) specific Synchronizers™.

During the Strain/Counterstrain technique, contact can be maintained on these Synchronizers™ and must also be maintained on the muscle. The Jones', or Advanced Strain/Counterstrain position is maintained while hand contact is maintained on these Synchronizers™. There are two (2) Synchronizers for improved muscle function which are appropriate to use with Strain and Counterstrain Technique; since the practitioner has only two hands, it is not possible to perform all of the following at once:

1. Attain and maintain the Strain and Counterstrain position.
2. Maintain hand contact on the muscle belly.
3. Maintain hand contact on the Process Center.
4. Maintain hand contact on the two (2) Synchronizers™.
5. Maintain hand contact on the access to the Mental Body.

   Note: #1 and #4 are the most important steps of the above.

There are a few options for practical application of all of the above. One option is as follows: The practitioner can maintain the Strain and Counterstrain position with hand contact on the muscle belly, while contacting the Process Center. When the fascial release is complete, the hand contact on the Process Center can be changed to hand contact on the first Synchronizer™. When this fascial release is complete, the hand contact can be changed to the second Synchronizer™. The second option is to have multiple hands performing this technique with hands contacting the Process Center, the two Synchronizers™, and the muscle belly at the same time.

The Synchronizers™ for Improved Muscle Function

SYNCHRONIZER™ #1

- Goal: Apparently To Release Tetanic Reflex to Motor End Plate.
- Location of Right and Left Synchronizers™: 3 cm's lateral to both L1 Transverse Processes.
- Procedure: To be used with Strain/Counterstrain positions. Maintain hand contact on muscle.

SYNCHRONIZER™ #2

- Goal: Apparently To Unlock Actin/Myosin Complex.
- Location of Left Synchronizer™: at interface of mesosigmoid/sigmoid colon.

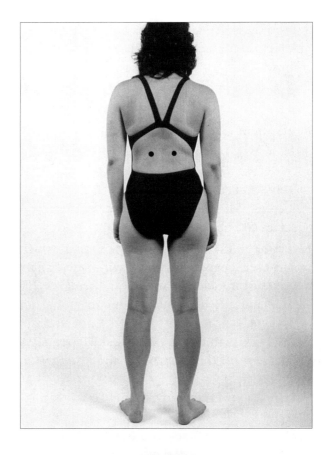

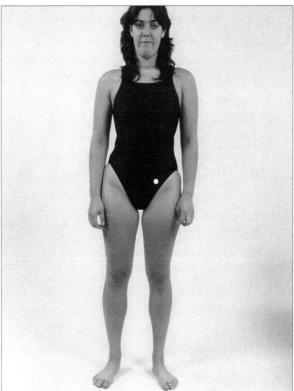

- Procedure: To be used with Strain/Counterstrain positions. Maintain hand contact on muscle.

(Biologic Analogs™, Copyright 1995 Lowen/Weiselfish-Giammatteo)

Neurologic Phenomenon for Treatment Integration (Weiselfish-Giammatteo)

1. Tonic and Anti-tonic Neuronal Activity Increase Muscle Tone with Strain/Counterstrain and 'Tonic Facilitation™.'

Left frontal and parietal lobes are *tonic,* which means their neuronal activity will predetermine the tone of muscles, ligaments and tendons. Increased muscle, ligament and tendon tone can be attained when the Strain and Counterstrain position is maintained while hand contact is maintained on the left frontal and left parietal regions.

    Step One: Maintain the Strain/Counterstrain Position.

    Step Two: Maintain hand contact on the left frontal and left parietal region of the cranium.

2. Tonic and Anti-tonic Neuronal Activity Decrease Muscle Tone with Strain/Counterstrain and 'Anti-Tonic De-Facilitation™.'

Right frontal and parietal lobes are *anti-tonic,* which means their neuronal activity will "tone-down" muscle, ligament, and tendon tension. Decreased muscle, ligament and tendon tone can be attained when the Strain and Counterstrain position is maintained while hand contact

is maintained on the right frontal and parietal regions.

    Step One: Maintain the Strain/Counterstrain position.

    Step Two: Maintain hand contact on the right frontal and right parietal region of the cranium.

3. Neurofascial Process™ for Agonistic and Antagonistic Neuronal Activity Treatment of the Neurologic Patient with Spasticity.

For the neurologic patient with hypertonicity (spasticity), *'antagonistic' neuronal activity* can be induced with right frontal and parietal hand contact. Antagonistic neuronal activity decreases the tone of agonist muscle.

    Step One: Maintain the Strain/Counterstrain position.

    Step Two: Maintain hand contact on the right frontal and right parietal region of the cranium.

4. Neurofascial Process™ for Agonistic and Antagonistic Neuronal Activity Treatment of the Neurologic Patient with Hypotonia.

For the neurologic patient with hypotonia, *'agonistic' neuronal activity* can be induced with left frontal and left parietal hand contact. Agonistic neuronal activity increases the tone of the agonist muscle.

    Step One: Maintain the Strain/Counterstrain position.

    Step Two: Maintain hand contact on the left frontal and left parietal region of the cranium.

CHAPTER 3

A HYPOTHETICAL MODEL

Decreasing the Hypertonicity of Protective Muscle Spasm and Spasticity with Strain and Counterstrain Technique and Advanced Strain and Counterstrain Technique

The musculofascialskeletal system receives most of the efferent outflow from the central nervous system; the largest portion of this efferent discharge exits the spinal cord via the ventral roots to the muscles. The musculofascialskeletal systems are also the source of much of the widespread, continuous, and variable sensory input to the CNS. This sensory feedback relayed from receptors in myofascial, visceral, articular components, and others, enters the spinal cord via the dorsal roots. This sensory reporting is routed to many centers throughout the central nervous system, including the cerebral cortex, the cerebellum, the brain stem, and the autonomic nervous system. This sensory input from the musculofascialskeletal body is extensive, intensive, and continuous, and is a dominant influence on the central nervous system.

The Premise

Disturbances in the sensory afferent input from the neuromusculoskeletal systems, whether diffuse or local, affect motor functions and other functions. This premise is a core concept, clinically significant for hypertonicity (protective muscle spasm and spasticity), the facilitated segment, and Structural Rehabilitation.

In 1947, Denslow stated a hypothesis which explained this concept:

> "(An) osteopathic lesion represents a facilitated segment of the spinal cord maintained in that state by impulses of *endogenous origin* entering the corresponding dorsal root. All structures receiving efferent nerve fibers from that segment are, therefore, potentially exposed to excessive excitation or inhibition."

The site of this *"endogenous origin"* is the *proprioceptors*, especially the muscle spindles. They are sensitive to musculofascialskeletal stresses. They are non adapting receptors, sustaining streams of impulses for as long as they are mechanically stimulated. Their influence is specific to the muscles acting on the affected joints, which are innervated by corresponding spinal segments.

The Myotatic Reflex Arc

The Myotatic Reflex Arc (also known as the stretch reflex arc, the monosynaptic reflex arc, and the gamma motor neuron loop), has long been considered as the basis of muscle tone. The components of this reflex arc include: the muscle fiber, which has the ability to contract, and to relax and elongate; the muscle spindle, the proprioceptor, which is responsive to length and velocity stretch; the gamma neuron which innervates the muscle spindle; the afferent neuron, which transcribes the information regarding stretch to the spinal cord; and the alpha motor neuron, which transcribes the impulse from the spinal cord to the muscle fiber, eliciting a muscle contraction.

The Muscle

The muscle is the focus of dysfunctional movement, when considering the hypertonicity of protective muscle spasm and spasticity. The muscle is active, self-energized, independent in motion and capable of developing great, widely variable, and rapidly changing forces. Other tissues are passively moved, immobilized, pushed, pulled, compressed, and altered in shape by those forces of muscular origin. Muscles *produce motion* by their contraction, but those same contractile forces also *oppose motion*. Contracting muscle absorbs momentum, and regulates, resists, retards, and arrests movement. Irvin Korr states that this energy-absorbing function of skeletal muscle is as important to the control of motion as its energy-imparting function. But the same cellular mechanisms are involved in these functions.

Joint mobility, range of motion, and ease of initiation of active motion are results of healthy muscle function. Limited capacity of muscles often appears to be the major impediment to mobility of a dysfunctional joint. Korr states that muscular resistance is not based on inextensibility, as with connective tissues, but on changes in the degree of activation and deactivation of the contractile tissue. The hypothetical cause for a muscle to increase or decrease its contraction and braking power is variations in impulse flow along the motor axons, the alpha neurons, which innervate the muscle. This neuronal impulse traffic varies with changing levels of excitation within the anterior horn cells, which change according to varying afferent input.

Proprioceptors

The muscle spindle, the proprioceptor within the muscle fibers which responds to stretch, is a basic component of the myotatic reflex arc, and has been implicated as a basic component of protective muscle spasm, and of spasticity. The proprioceptors are the sensory end organs that signal physical changes in musculofascialskeletal tissues. The three main categories of proprioceptors are sensitive to joint position and motion, to tendon tension, and to muscle length.

The *joint receptors* are located in joint capsules and ligaments; they report joint motion and position. The Ruffini endings in the capsules report direction, velocity of motion, and position very accurately. These joint receptors do not appear to have significant influence on

motor activity via the stretch reflex arc, although this premise is presently under investigation.

The *Golgi tendon receptors* are located in tendons close to the musculotendinous junction. A pull on the tendon causes discharge of impulses into the spinal cord via afferent fibers. This pull is usually exerted by active contraction of the muscle. The tendon endings are responsive to changes in force, not in length. When the muscle contracts against a load, or fixed object, or against the contraction of antagonistic muscles as in spasticity and protective muscle spasm, the discharge of the tendon endings is in proportion to the tension that is developed. The afferent input from the Golgi tendon varies with the tension exerted by the muscle on the tendon, regardless of the muscle length. The discharges of the tendon endings enter the spinal cord by dorsal root fibers, where they excite *inhibitory* interneurons that synapse with motor neurons controlling the same muscle. The effect of their discharge is inhibitory; it tends to oppose the further development of tension by the muscle.

The Muscle Spindle

The *muscle spindles* are complex. Each spindle has two kinds of sensory endings with different reflex influences, each with its own motor innervation. Spindles are scattered throughout each muscle, the quantity varying according to the function of the muscle and the delicacy of its control. The greater the spindle density, the finer the control. The complex anatomy and physiology of the muscle spindles is well documented in the literature.

Spindles are within the muscle itself, surrounded by muscle fibers, arranged in parallel with them and attached to them at both ends. Stretching the muscle causes stretch of the spindle; shortening of the muscle slackens the spindle. Each spindle, enclosed in a connective tissue sheath, about 3 mm long, has several thin muscle fibers. These are the *intrafusal fibers*. The larger and more powerful *extrafusal fibers* comprise the bulk of the muscle. The intrafusal fibers are attached to the sheath at each end. *The intrafusal muscle fibers are innervated by gamma motor neuron fibers* originating in the ventral horn, passing through the ventral root. *The alpha motor neurons supply innervation to the extrafusal muscle fibers.*

The sensory endings of the spindle are in close relation to the central, nucleated, noncontractile portion of the intrafusal fibers. This sensory ending, called the *primary ending*, is wound around the intrafusal fibers, described as the *annulospiral ending*. Secondary, *flowerspray endings* occur on either side of the primary ending and are connected to thinner myelinated axons. Both are sensitive to stretch of the central portion of the spindle.

There is a static and a dynamic response to stretch by the muscle: static is proportional to muscle length; dynamic is proportional to the rate of change in muscle length. The intrafusal muscle fiber is relatively elastic: the IA afferent endings, which innervate the primary nerve endings, end here. Therefore, the IA fiber has a dynamic and a static response to stretch. The group II afferent fibers, which innervate the secondary endings, end on the small nuclear chain fibers. This is at the area of the heart of the myofibril striations of the intrafusal fibers: a less elastic, stiffer area. Therefore there is only a static response to stretch which is proportional to muscle length. Since these fibers have no dynamic response, they will not carry central nervous system feedback regarding the velocity of the stretch.

The *primary endings*, or *annulospiral endings*, *respond to change in muscle length.* When the muscle is stretched beyond its resting length, the spindle is stretched, causing the primary and secondary endings to fire at increased frequencies in proportion to the degree of stretch. Shortening of the muscle, whether by its own contraction or by passive approximation of its attachments, slows the discharge proportionately, and may even silence it.

The spindle, an essential feedback mechanism by which the muscle is controlled, continually reports back to the central nervous system. The feedback from the primary endings of each spindle is conveyed by dorsal root fiber directly, that is, monosynaptically, to the alpha motoneurons of the same muscle. This afferent discharge of the spindle results in excitation of the alpha motor neurons of the same muscle. How does this occur? *When a muscle is stretched, it is reflexly stimulated by its spindles to contract*, and thereby resists stretching. This protective reflex response is at the spinal cord level of the same spinal segment. The *protective shortening of the muscle decreases the afferent discharge*, and thus reduces the excitation of the alpha motor neurons, *causing relaxation and lengthening of the muscle.*

The muscle spindle causes the muscle to resist change in length in either direction. The spindle is the sensory component of the stretch, reflex arc, or myotatic reflex arc. It is important in maintenance of posture. The intrafusal muscle fibers influence spindle discharge. Their ends are anchored, and contraction of these intrafusal fibers stretches the middle portion in which the sensory endings are situated, increasing their discharge. *The effect of intrafusal contraction on the sensory endings is indistinguishable from the effect produced by stretch of the extrafusal fibers.* The two effects are cumulative. At any lengthening of the muscle, intrafusal contraction would increase the spindle discharge; stretch of the muscle while the intrafusal fibers are contracted produces a more intense spindle discharge than when the intrafusal fibers are at rest or less contracted.

The Gamma Neuron

The gamma neuron, a component of the myotatic reflex arc, (or gamma motor neuron loop), innervates the muscle spindle, is affected by dysfunction within the neuromusculoskeletal system, and is controlled by the brain and supraspinal neurons. The function of the gamma neurons is to control contraction of the intrafusal fibers, the frequency of the spindle discharge at a given muscle length, and the sensitivity or change in that frequency per millimeter change in length. The higher the gamma activity, the larger the spindle response; the higher the spindle discharge at a given muscle length, the shorter the length of muscle at which a given impulse frequency is generated. *This explains the threshold to stretch of the spindle.*

The *gamma neurons, also known as "fusimotor" neurons* are small in size and their axons are thin. Fusimotor innervation by the gamma fibers comprise one-third of the ventral root outflow from the spinal cord. Alpha-to-gamma and extrafusal-to-intrafusal relationships regulate the activity of skeletal muscles. *The higher the spindle discharge, the greater the reflex contraction of the muscle.* What that muscle contraction accomplishes depends on the other forces acting on the joints crossed by that muscle. Generally, the greater the contraction, the more the muscle shortens and moves the joint, and the more it resists being stretched in the opposite direction.

Gamma Bias

Normal resting conditions of gamma activity maintain a tonic afferent discharge from the spindle. This is the *gamma bias*. This maintains the alpha motor neurons in a moderately facilitated state, and the muscles in low-grade tonic contraction at their resting lengths. Thus, people are not flaccid and hypotonic, but maintain some muscle tone. Gamma activity may be turned up or down. The higher the gamma activity, because of its influence on the excitatory spindle discharge, the more forceful the muscle's contraction and the greater its resistance to being lengthened. During high gamma activity, or *gamma gain*, the spindle may elicit contrac-

tion when the muscle is already shorter than its resting length. If the increased gamma gain is sustained, the muscle contraction is maintained. This is muscle spasm.

The sensory endings of the spindle are stimulated by mechanical distortion, whether caused by contraction of the intrafusal fibers or by stretch of the main muscle, or both. The spindle in effect reports length *relative* to that of the intrafusal fibers. The greater the disparity in length, the greater the discharge and the greater the contraction of the muscle. Increase in intrafusal-extrafusal disparity increases the afferent discharge, which results in a contractile response of the extrafusal fibers, which in turn tends to reduce the disparity and to silence the spindle. *The greater the gamma activity, the more the muscle must shorten before the spindle is turned back down to resting discharge and normal gamma bias. The central nervous system can elicit and precisely control gamma bias.*

There is always some activity around this myotatic reflex arc. There is a certain *gamma bias: a certain level of activity along the gamma neuron which results in a resting threshold to stretch of the muscle spindle, controlled by the central nervous system.* Evidently the gamma neuron is inhibited by supraspinal structures. When there is a cortical lesion, the suppressor areas of the brain which inhibit the gamma neuron are damaged. The inhibition process via the medial reticular formation is affected. An increased level of activity within the myotatic reflex arc occurs because of the resultant increase in gamma bias. Gamma bias is no longer normal, due to disinhibition of the central nervous system. The result is spasticity, which is hypertonicity, plus other characteristics of the syndrome of spasticity. The gamma gain and the hyperactivity of the myotatic reflex arc result in the hypertonicity of protective muscle spasm and spasticity.

The Afferent Neuron

Whenever the muscle spindle is stimulated, via stretch stimulus, that information passes along the afferent neuron into the posterior horn of the spinal cord of that spinal segment. Some of this sensory input is distributed throughout the central nervous system. Much of the sensory input passes as discharge along the same afferent neuron to the anterior horn of that same spinal segment. In the ventral horn, this discharge passes across the synapse to the neuron of the alpha motor nerve, and passes along the length of the alpha motor neuron axon, to the muscle fiber. When the muscle fiber receives the impulse, it contracts and shortens.

Neuromusculoskeletal Dysfunction and the Hyperactive Myotatic Reflex Arc

This hypothetical model expands on Denslow's and Korr's hypothesis of the Osteopathic lesion, in order to provide a model which explains the results of Manual Therapy for treatment of neuromusculoskeletal dysfunction. These results include increased resting muscle length, increased joint mobility, and increased ranges of motion.

A Hypothetical Model

Envision a cross section of the spinal cord at the level of C5. The embryologic segment of C5 spinal cord innervates certain tissues and structures. Among these tissues and structures are: the supraspinatus muscle, the deltoid muscle, the infraspinatus muscle, the subscapularis muscle, the biceps muscle (C5,6), and more. When there is dysfunction in one or more of the tissues and structures which are innervated by the C5 embryologic segment, there is resultant increase in gamma gain, and protective muscle spasm of the musculature innervated by that same C5 segment.

Neuromusculoskeletal Dysfunction Causes Afferent Gain; Afferent Gain Causes Alpha Gain

When a person has a supraspinatus tendinitis, the brain is apprized of this status. The person perceives pain at the shoulder. The pain is generic: the person does not know that the pain is the result of a supraspinatus dysfunction. *The afferent neuron, bringing the sensory information about this dysfunction to the spinal cord, will pass this information as excessive and high frequency discharge.* This is similar to the excessive and high frequency discharge of gamma gain, but it is "afferent gain". The afferent neuron from the supraspinatus muscle and tendon will pass the sensory information along the afferent neuron as increased afferent gain, which enters the spinal cord via the dorsal roots and posterior horn of C5 spinal segment.

This excessive and high frequency discharge is distributed throughout the central nervous system: cortex, brain stem, up one or more spinal segments, down one or more spinal segments, across to the opposite side of the spinal cord, and more. Some of this excessive and high frequency discharge is also passed along the afferent neuron to the anterior horn. At the ventral horn, the excessive and high frequency discharge passes across the synapse and affects the alpha motor neuron which innervates the supraspinatus muscle. This same excessive and high frequency discharge passes along the length of the alpha motor neuron which innervates the supraspinatus muscle.

This excessive and high frequency discharge, passing down the length of the alpha motor neuron to the muscle fiber, is *alpha gain*, or the increase in discharge and activity of the alpha motor neuron. When an impulse reaches the muscle fiber, the muscle fiber contracts and shortens. If excessive and too frequent discharge passes along the alpha motor neuron, the muscle fiber will go into a state of contraction which is sustained by the continuous volley of impulses. The muscle fiber, the supraspinatus, can no longer voluntarily relax and elongate. This is the model of *protective muscle spasm* of the supraspinatus which results from a supraspinatus tendinitis dysfunction.

If there is a supraspinatus tendinitis, the supraspinatus muscle will go into a state of protective muscle spasm, contracted and shortened, incapable of attaining full resting length due to an inability to relax and elongate. The supraspinatus crosses the glenohumeral joint. The joint surfaces will become approximated, resulting in joint hypomobility and limitations in ranges of motion.

Gamma Gain: Increased Sensitivity of the Muscle Spindle and Decreased Threshold to Stretch

The excessive and high frequency discharge which is passed into the alpha motor neuron in the anterior horn is also passed into the gamma motor neuron. Alpha and gamma signals are linked and coordinated in the spinal segment. The gamma motor neuron passes this excessive and high frequency discharge down to the muscle spindle. The muscle spindle is now hyper-innervated. Therefore, the sensitivity of the spindle to stretch is increased; the threshold of the muscle spindle to stretch will be decreased. The spindle will be "hyperactivated", and will react to smaller stretch, and lower velocity of stretch, than before the supraspinatus tendinitis was present. There is a facilitation of the my-otatic reflex arc: *the stretch reflex arc is hyperactive.* This phenomenon is called a "*facilitated segment.*"

The Facilitated Segment and Efferent Gain of Alpha and Gamma Neurons

Increased efferent gain is characteristic of the facilitated segment. The alpha motor neurons which innervate the supraspinatus muscle fibers are not the only neurons to exit from the anterior horn of C5 embryologic segment. The other alpha neurons, for example, those which inner-

vate the subscapularis, infraspinatus, deltoid, and biceps (C5,6), can also pass the excessive and high frequency discharge accumulating in the ventral horn, as the condition of the supraspinatus tendinitis becomes more severe and more chronic. This excessive and high frequency discharge in the anterior horn, when sufficient to influence the other neurons, will pass along those other alpha motor neurons innervated by the same C5 spinal segment. *Thus there is a potential and tendency for protective muscle spasm of all the muscles innervated by that same C5 embryologic segment which innervates the supraspinatus. This situation becomes exacerbated as the tendinitis becomes more severe and more chronic.*

The gamma neurons, which innervate the intrafusal muscle fibers of the muscle spindles of all the muscles innervated by this same C5 embryologic segment, can also pass this excessive and high frequency discharge, as the dysfunction becomes more severe and more chronic. *As a result, the sensitivity of these spindles to stretch is increased, and the threshold of stretch of all the muscle spindles innervated by this spinal segment is decreased.* The potential for protective muscle spasm and dysfunction is exacerbated. All these muscle cross the glenohumeral joint, therefore the approximation of the humeral head in the glenoid fossa, the joint hypomobility, the disturbance of articular balance, and the limitations in ranges of motion are exacerbated.

Somatovisceral Reflex Arcs

Neurons exiting the spinal cord innervate more than muscle spindles and muscle fibers. They also provide innervation of viscera via the autonomic nervous system. For example, L1 innervates the cecum. If a patient with a history of an appendectomy has scarring within the lower right abdominal cavity, this information will be passed as sensory feedback via the afferent neurons to the central nervous system. Afferent neurons, passing this information as excessive and high frequency discharge, enter the spinal cord via the posterior horn of L1. From here the sensory information is distributed throughout the central nervous system. Some of the information is also relayed to the anterior horn of this same L1 embryologic segment. All the alpha motor neurons which are innervated by L1 embryologic segments can potentially pass this excessive and high frequency discharge, which is accumulating in L1 anterior horn, and can pass this hyperactivity along the alpha motor neurons, which would result in protective muscle spasm of the muscle fibers innervated by that same L1 segment. Also, all the muscle spindles innervated by the gamma neurons from this L1 segment which could potentially pass the excessive and high frequency discharge will be affected, so that the threshold to stretch of all these muscle spindles would be decreased. This facilitated segment at L1, the result of dysfunctional tissue surrounding the cecum, may cause somatic dysfunction of the pelvis and hip joint region because of the sustained contraction of the muscles crossing those joints.

The Self-Perpetuating Hyperactive Reflex Arc

Occasionally, the supraspinatus tendinitis may be so severe and so chronic that healing of the tendinitis with effective Manual Therapy intervention is not sufficient to decrease the hyperactivity of the stretch reflex arc. The hyperactivity of the myotatic reflex arc has become self-perpetuating. There remains some excessive and high frequency discharge passed along the neurons within this gamma motor neuron loop, in spite of the Manual Therapy which "cured" the supraspinatus tendinitis. There is an apparent disinhibition of this hyperactive reflex arc: the increased gamma gain is maintained in spite of the decrease in afferent gain. The gamma gain is increased, as it is in cases of spasticity, when the brain and supraspinal structures are affected in the neurologic patient. The inhibition of gamma

activity by the suppressor areas of the brain does not appear to be effective in maintaining a normal gamma bias. The hypertonicity of the muscle spindles and the fibers is maintained. Is this situation possible? It is this situation which occurs when there is a cortical lesion, for example, with the hemiplegic: a self-perpetuating hyperactive reflex arc due to disinhibition of supraspinal structures.

In these cases, it is necessary to address this self-perpetuating hyperactive reflex arc as a primary problem. Initially, this myotatic reflex arc became hyperactive secondary to the supraspinatus tendinitis. Now, due to a chronic and severe supraspinatus dysfunction, it is a primary self-perpetuating problem. A Manual Therapy technique developed by Lawrence Jones, D.O., called Strain and Counterstrain Technique, appears to successfully "shut down" the hyperactivity within this reflex arc. In the case of a self-perpetuating protective muscle spasm of this supraspinatus muscle, the technique would result in an apparent reduction and arrest of the proprioceptor activity of the muscle spindles of the supraspinatus muscle fibers. There is a decrease in the gamma gain. This technique is performed by shortening the muscle fibers and spindles of the muscle (for example, the supraspinatus muscle), while putting a stretch on the Golgi tendon of the antagonist of this muscle. Korr and others have provided evidence that shortening of the muscle spindle, together with the stretch on the Golgi tendon of the antagonist muscle, results in a decrease and even an arrest in the gamma neuronal and proprioceptor activity. There is apparently a general decrease of this excessive and high frequency discharge passed around this hyperactive reflex arc. This technique results in an effective elimination of protective muscle spasm of the muscle treated, with a relaxation and elongation of the resting muscle fibers. There are increases in joint mobility and ranges of motion as a result of the elimination of the protective muscle spasm. The mechanism of correction is not known. This author speculates that the shut-down of the hyperactivity of the muscle spindle will decrease the gamma gain to a normal gamma bias, which will facilitate a linking and a coordination between the inhibition process of the central nervous system and the myotatic reflex arc. This linking process is a neurophysiologic phenomenon which requires 90 seconds.

Spasticity and the Myotatic Reflex Arc: A Hypothetical Model

The Therapist with an understanding of spasticity can utilize this hypothetical model to explain the results of Manual Therapy on reducing hypertonicity in the neurologic patient. The abnormal muscle tone and coordination in the neurologic patient are due to the release of abnormal postural reflexes. The normal postural reflex mechanism consists mainly of three groups of automatic reactions. These include the righting reactions, which attain and maintain the position of the head in space (face vertical and mouth horizontal) and its symmetrical relationship with the trunk. The equilibrium reactions attain and maintain balance during activities to prevent falling. Reactions which automatically adapt muscles to postural changes in the trunk and extremities are the third group included in this category.

The described postural reflex mechanisms are necessary for voluntary functional activity. They provide normal postural tone via central nervous system activation of muscles in patterns, involving large groups of muscles. Normal reciprocal interaction of muscles allows stabilization of proximal body parts; this allows distal mobility. Automatic protective reactions, such as righting and equilibrium reactions, in gross movement patterns, are the background for voluntary functional activity. Associated reactions as described by Walshe are tonic reflexes; they are released postural reactions in

musculature deprived of voluntary control. In the neurologic patient, these associated reactions produce a widespread increase of spasticity throughout the affected side.

Spasticity is considered a major affliction, and although the neurophysiology of spasticity has been considered in detail by several researchers, there is no unanimous agreement of its definition. The most commonly discussed characteristics of spasticity include: 1. exaggerated stretch reflexes; 2. tendon (phasic) reflexes with a increased threshold to tapping; 3. increased response by tapped muscles; 4. increased response of tonic stretch reflexes; 5. clonus which may be induced.

Characteristics of Spasticity

- increased passive/resistance to stretch
- clonus
- flexor spasm
- alternating flexor and extensor spasm
- overflow
- hyperreflexia
- extensor synergy
- flexor synergy
- spastic equinovarus
- co-contraction
- dyssynergy
- clasp-knife response
- flexor withdrawal
- spastic gait
- associated movements
- irradiation
- spastic paraplegia
- spastic hemiplegia
- "alpha" spasticity
- "gamma" spasticity
- increased tone
- abnormal tone
- excessive or increased motor unit activity
- alternating clonus

Studies performed by Sherrington on decerebrate cats were important in providing a useful animal model for the conception of pathogenic factors in spasticity. The motor manifestations were found to be those of human spasticity. Sherrington concluded that decerebrate rigidity is reflexly maintained by the extrapyramidal tract, which is phylogenetically newer than the pyramidal system. He concluded that the muscle proprioceptors, which are the muscle spindles, are responsible for this decerebrate rigidity.

The gamma motor neuron loop, and the gamma motor system discussed in this Learner's Workbook, were first described by Leskell in 1945. As described, it is assumed that the gamma system controls the length and velocity of the spindles' primary endings, and the length sensitivity of the secondary endings. Gamma activity maintains appropriate spindle discharge at all muscle lengths during movement. This phenomenon is also true for the patient with spasticity.

As described above, the muscle spindles lie parallel to, and are attached to, the extrafusal muscle fibers. Passive muscle stretch causes spindle discharge from the primary endings. This results in a depolarization of alpha motor neurons until muscle contraction occurs. This is via a negative feedback control circuit, called the monosynaptic reflex arc, or stretch reflex arc, or myotatic reflex arc, or gamma motor neuron loop, to counteract changes in muscle length, due to passive stretch.

There is dual innervation of the muscle by the alpha:motor neuron to the extrafusal muscle fibers, and by the gamma neurons to the intrafusal muscle fiber of the muscle spindle. Their motor neurons are coordinated. Influenced by brain impulses, they fire at appropriate rates to attain smooth movements. The neurologic patient with a brain lesion no longer has these signals linked and coordinated.

Spasticity is considered the release of inhibition of the gamma neuron system, normally imposed by extrapyramidal impulses; the result of this disinhibition is the hyperactivity of the gamma neuron system, and the excessive and high frequency discharge of the gamma motor neurons. Therefore, there is an excessive and high frequency discharge from the primary endings of the muscle spindles. Thus, within the monosynaptic reflex arc, the alpha motor neurons will also have high frequency firing. The result is hyperactivity, hypertonicity, and spasticity, of the skeletal muscle.

Apparently, the alpha motor neuron system is rarely released from higher inhibitory control. Occasionally, brain lesions disrupt their supraspinal inhibition. In these cases, interrupting the gamma-spindle loop will not reduce the spasticity. Typically, brain lesions result in disinhibition of the gamma neuron system.

The lateral reticular formation appears to be a major source of facilitation of the gamma motor neurons; their supraspinal inhibition appears to synapse from the medial reticular formation. Although the lateral reticular formation is inherently active, neurons from the medial reticular formation need impulses from suppressor areas in order to release the impulses which exert an inhibitory effect upon the lower motor neurons. Therefore, *brain lesions which destroy these suppressor areas reduce the inhibitory drive of the medial reticular formation. This lack of inhibition results in an imbalance of the system: there is excessive facilitation to gamma motor neurons. Signs of hyperactive muscle spindles and spasticity appear. Normal gamma bias cannot be maintained. Increased gamma gain results.*

Although the gamma neurons are smaller than the alpha neurons, both are located in the ventral horns of the spinal cord. These smaller gamma neurons, which terminate on the intrafusal fibers as trail endings and plate endings, need less excitatory input to discharge than do the larger neurons. Without sufficient input to fire, the alpha neurons can remain quiet; gamma neurons are tonically firing. This is the gamma bias. A muscle spindle with increased gamma bias (gamma gain) will be more responsive to stretch than a passive spindle. Therefore the intrafusal fibers innervated by gamma neurons, with gamma gain, are in a active state of contraction.

If indeed the sensitivity of the primary and secondary sensory endings is a function of the level of the gamma bias, then with high gamma bias, or gamma gain, there will be a high frequency discharge from these sensory endings of the muscle spindle.

There are static and dynamic gamma motor neurons; 3/4 of these are static. Different areas of the brain control static and dynamic gamma activity. Thus the brain lesion location will define the dysfunction as static, dynamic, or both.

Patients with spasticity may have similar motor signs, but their underlying neural mechanisms differ. The final common pathway is the alpha motor neuron. *Hypertonicity as found in the spastic state is a reflection of the excessive excitatory drive to these alpha neurons, transmitted to them via the hyperactive monosynaptic reflex arc, due to release of inhibition causing excessive gamma gain.* This is evidenced by the hyperactive tonic stretch reflexes: upon passive stretch to a limb, resistance is encountered. The strength of this resistance depends upon the velocity of the movement: slower motion, decreased resistance. This reflex appears to be an objective measure of dynamic gamma motor nerve involvement. Since most spastic muscles do not respond to static stretch, the static gamma nervous system is possibly not the site of excitatory excess. Tonic stretch reflexes elicit exaggerated responses only after exceeding certain velocity threshold, after which the response is proportional to the velocity of the movement.

The Group II afferents, which innervate the secondary endings that respond only to static stretch, synapse on two types of neurons: those which inhibit extensor motor neurons, and those which excite flexor motor neurons. Therefore the tonic stretch reflex is typically suppressed in extensor muscles and enhanced in the flexor muscles.

Hyperactive phasic stretch reflexes is another characteristic of spasticity. The monosynaptic reflex arc is as follows: the tendon is tapped; the muscle spindle is thus stretched; primary endings then fire; action potentials travel to the spinal cord via 1A afferents; alpha motor neurons are then excited; there is a muscle contraction. With the phasic response, there is no dependency upon velocity sensitivity of the primary endings.

These hyperactive stretch reflex arcs impede voluntary control. Agonist function is impeded by the hyperactivity of the antagonist and dysfunction of the agonist. Sahrman and Norton gave evidence through electromyography that primary impairment of movement in the hemiplegic patient is not due to this antagonist spasticity, but due to limited and prolonged recruitment of agonist contraction. They state that these muscles are slower to attain maximal EMG levels, and do not elicit the quantity or frequency of motor unit discharge produced by normal individuals.

There is an intimate relationship between spasticity and movement in the neurologic patient: lack of voluntary movement appears largely due to spasticity. The weakness of muscles, documented by Sahrman and Norton, may not be real, but relative to the opposition of their spastic antagonists and the gamma gain of the muscle itself. *Reduce the spasticity and these weak muscles often show increased power.* Therefore, the techniques used to test muscle strength in clinical orthopedic disorders are not appropriate for the neurologic patient because of the compromise of muscle control. Muscle testing in non-central nervous system lesions depends upon the ability to simultaneously contract the agonist and relax the antagonist. The muscle function must be independent of stretch and rate of stretch.

These muscle tests also rely on the patient's ability to be indifferent to the posture of the limb and body. But the associated movements in the neurologic patient which also cause the impairment of selectivity of movement are primitive, stereotypic synergies: patterns of mass flexion and extension, these synergies are not pathological movements, but normal humans can perform relatively independently of these patterns. These synergies are the same as those found in the primitive withdrawal and thrust reflexes. But a reflex is an involuntary reaction to a sensory stimulus; the primitive pattern response is a voluntary action. It is initiated when the neurologic patient wants to perform an act. No sensory stimulus is needed to elicit these patterns.

The effects of these repetitive primitive patterns are severe: they could almost become permanent changes in movement patterns. Although the neural mechanism is not clearly understood, it is known that the repetition of movement patterns can cause long term alteration of performance. The abnormal postures and muscle activity will cause structural changes in joints and muscles. Hyperactive muscles will hypertrophy; inactive muscles will atrophy. Post-tetanic potentiation will occur: central nervous system synapses exposed to repetitive activity present a long lasting pre-synaptic facilitation. The repetitive action caused by these recurring patterns could induce an exaggerated response in the nerve to synthesize, mobilize, and transmit neurotransmitters. Repetitive activity has shown increased amplitude in the excitatory post-synaptic potential, when evoked by single nerve impulse repetition. This post- tetanic potentiation may aggravate the spasticity. The high frequency discharge of the IA fibers may cause post-tetanic potentiation at the monosynaptic connections of the alpha neurons.

In the neurologic patient, the positive sup- porting reaction is also released from supraspinal control; when combined with extensor spasticity of the leg it becomes a severe spastic response. This positive supporting reaction is the static modification of the spinal extensor thrust described by Sherrington: a brief extensor reaction, evoked by a stimulus of sudden pressure to the pads of the foot, and affecting all the extensor muscles of the limb, with relaxation of their antagonists. Adequate stimulus for this reaction includes: proprioceptive stimulus by stretching foot intrinsic muscles, and exteroceptive stimulus by contacting pads of the foot with the ground. The reaction is characterized by simultaneous contraction of flexors and extensors, so that joints are fixated.

Brain lesions can affect not only the gamma and alpha systems, and the release of primitive patterns of movement, but also the interneurons in the intermediate grey matter of the spinal cord. In the animal model, flexor withdrawal cannot be elicited. To elicit flexor withdrawal during extensor spasticity, the flexor motor neurons must be excited, while hyperactive extensors are inhibited. There is a polysynaptic reflex arc with one neuron to excite flexors and another to inhibit extensors. In brain stem transsections there is depression of this reciprocal inhibition.

Manual Therapy for Treatment of Neuromusculoskeletal Dysfunction and Spasticity

The reduction of excessive gamma activity is the basic rationale which explains why Manual Therapy reduces spasticity in the neurologic patient. Manual Therapy which is effective in treatment of neuromusculoskeletal dysfunction will typically result in: reducing the hyperactivity and gamma gain; decreasing the primitive patterns of movement; strengthening voluntary controls. *The same hyperactive Myotatic Reflex Arc implicated in protective muscle spasm is associated with the hypertonicity component of spasticity*. Due to brain lesions and lesions of supraspinal structures, there is an apparent hyperactivity of this reflex arc secondary to a disinhibition of the gamma neuron system.

Pre-injury Neuromusculoskeletal Dysfunction in the Neurologic Patient

Human beings typically present with varying degrees of neuromusculoskeletal dysfunction somewhere in the body. Statistics indicate that 8 of 10 Americans suffer back pain during their lifetimes. This pain probably is the result of neuromusculoskeletal dysfunction: biomechanical dysfunction and joint hypomobility; protective muscle spasm; connective tissue dysfunction; and more. It may be assumed that there is pre-existing neuromusculoskeletal dysfunction and protective muscle spasm in the neurologic patient, prior to the central nervous system insult. The hyperactive Myotatic Reflex Arc is present due to neuromusculoskeletal dysfunction in all patient populations: clinical orthopedic, sports medicine, chronic pain, pediatric, and neurologic.

The gamma neuron, with increased gamma gain, and the muscle spindle, is the seat of protective muscle spasm and spasticity. According to this model, normalization and healing of neuromusculoskeletal dysfunction with effective Manual Therapy should result in decrease of excessive and high frequency discharge within this hyperactive myotatic reflex arc in the neurologic patient population, as in other patient populations. *Effective Manual Therapy techniques, which correct neuromusculoskeletal dysfunction, achieve decreased hypertonicity, whether in the form of protective muscle spasm or spasticity,* for the orthopedic and the neurologic patient. In the case of a self perpetuating hyperactive reflex arc, associated with primary hypertonicity, utilization of Strain and Counterstrain Techniques results in a decrease in proprioceptor activity and a decrease in the

hyperactivity within that reflex arc. This contributes to a decrease of the hypertonicity of spasticity as well as a decrease of the hypertonicity of primary protective muscle spasm.

Effect of Manual Therapy on Central Nervous System Activity of the Neurologic Patient

Afferent information of sensory input is distributed throughout the central nervous system, to the brain and the spinal cord. Manual Therapy which corrects neuromusculoskeletal dysfunction achieves a decrease in general afferent gain. Therefore, a decrease in the efferent gain which is affecting the muscle fibers innervated by other spinal segments can be expected. Utilization of Manual Therapy to correct and heal neuromusculoskeletal dysfunction results in more than the decrease of protective muscle spasm of the muscles innervated by the segment that innervates the dysfunctional tissue or structure. *There is a resultant decrease in the severity of the protective muscle spasm in muscles innervated by other segments of the spinal cord as well. There will be a resultant decrease in the general level of spasticity also.*

Utilization of Strain and Counterstrain Technique to decrease and arrest the inappropriate proprioceptor activity of the muscle spindle, and to eliminate the hyperactivity within the reflex arc of a muscle, will result in a decrease in general efferent gain as well. Therefore, the protective muscle spasm of all the muscles innervated by that same segment, as well as muscles innervated by other segments, will diminish. For the neurologic patient, the general level of spasticity of the musculature surrounding the treated muscle will also decrease. Utilization of Manual Therapy Techniques will beneficially affect spasticity.

The facilitated segment as described above is a concept basic to the philosophy of Structural Rehabilitation for the neurologic patient. The author has presented a model. If research discovers new information, which negates this model, then a new hypothesis for a new model will be needed. Structural Rehabilitation for the neurologic population does not require a hypothetical model for the successful integration of this work for improved rehabilitation results.

Summary: A Conceptual Model for the Neurologic Patient

- The muscle spindle innervation by the gamma neuron.
- Inhibitory control of the gamma neuron by the central nervous system.
- Afferent Gain: excessive and inappropriate sensory input into the spinal cord due to neuromusculoskeletal dysfunction.
- Distribution of excessive and high frequency discharge throughout the central nervous system: hyperactivity of the central nervous system.
- Alpha Gain: excessive and high frequency discharge affecting the alpha motor neuron innervation of the muscle fiber.
- Hyperinnervated sarcomere: a contracted and shortened muscle due to alpha gain.
- Hyperactive myotatic reflex arc: afferent gain; alpha gain; gamma gain.
- Protective muscle spasm: a hyperactive myotatic reflex arc causing sustained contracted and shortened sarcomeres. A basis of pathokinesiology: muscles crossing the joints will cause approximation of joint surfaces, joint hypomobility and limitations of ranges of motion.
- Articular Balance: imbalance in the resting position of articular surfaces due to protective muscle spasm in muscles crossing the joint and exerting pathologic forces on the bones at muscle insertion and origin.
- Gamma Gain: due to excessive and high frequency discharge in the ventral horn; resulting in inappropriate and excessive proprioceptor activity.

- Hypersensitivity: The sensitivity to stretch of the muscle spindle is increased. The threshold of tolerance of the muscle spindle to stimuli and stretch and dysfunction is lowered. A smaller stimulus can activate the facilitated segment.
- The Facilitated Segment: efferent gain of the gamma and alpha neurons potentiates protective muscle spasm of all muscles innervated by that segment.
- Hyperactivity: Not only is the segment hypersensitive with a decreased threshold to become more activated, but the segment overreacts to stimuli. The excessive and high frequency discharge in that segment will influence every tissue and structure innervated by that segment. Central nervous system inhibitory effects on the segment are less effective.
- Protective Muscle Spasm of the musculature innervated by that segment.
- Protective Muscle Spasm of musculature innervated by other segments.
- Dysautonomia: Sympathetic ganglia are affected by the excessive and high frequency discharge of the spinal segment. The threshold to "fight and flight" and stress is lowered. Healing is affected. Visceral function, lymphatic system function, connective tissue function, immune system function is affected. There is a correlating attempt for parasympathetic nervous system balancing, which affects digestive and cardiovascular function.
- Dystrophic Effect: Irwin Korr discovered the trophic effect of the neuron which manufactures and transports protein to vitalize the end organs: e.g. the muscle fiber. This function is affected when the neuron is "facilitated." The reduction of this trophic effect is dystrophy, which affects all end organs.
- Defacilitation: can be achieved with Manual Therapy: 1) by correcting and healing the neuromusculoskeletal dysfunction, 2) by reducing and arresting inappropriate proprioceptor activity and the self-perpetuating

hyperactive reflex arc with Strain and Counterstrain Technique, 3) by Manual and Cranial Therapy to defacilitate the facilitated segment and the spinal cord.

- Corrective Kinesiology: As a result of the relaxation and elongation of the muscle fiber achieved with effective Manual Therapy, there is improved articular balance, with a more normal resting position of articular surfaces. There is decreased muscle resistance to movement, increased joint mobility, increased ranges of motion, and improved posture for the orthopedic and the neurologic patient.

CHAPTER 4

APPLICATION

How to Perform Advanced Strain and Counterstrain Technique

A Note of Caution

Use the "Mechanical Model." Do not use the Tender Point. The autonomic nervous system is especially susceptible to stimulation by pressure on the tender points!

At Regional Physical Therapy we use the Mechanical Model/Corrective Kinesiologic Model with Jones' Strain and Counterstrain Technique. During more than a decade of research, we have discovered that many persons do not have "normal" sensory perception; the Tender Points may not reflect the true status of hypertonicity of the patient. We also discovered that stimulation of the Tender Points of Advanced Strain and Counterstrain Technique can set off a long-term treatment reaction which is difficult to contain.

De-Facilitated Fascial Release™

De-Facilitated Fascial Release™ (Weiselfish-Giammatteo) is the phenomenon of "tissue unwinding" which occurs when there is "de-facilitation." De-facilitation is the decrease of afferent and efferent discharge. Strain and Counterstrain Technique and Advanced Strain and Counterstrain Technique cause de-facilitation.

Maintain the precise position of the Strain and Counterstrain Technique or Advanced Strain and Counterstrain Technique throughout the duration of tissue tension transformation.

How to Perform a De-Facilitated Fascial Release™

1. After one-minute duration of the Advanced Strain and Counterstrain technique, continue to maintain the precise position of the technique.
2. Maintain this position precisely, without any movement added, until there is no sensation of movement, or any other sensation.
3. The De-Facilitated Fascial Release™ is the tissue "unwinding" which occurs secondary to the elimination and/or decrease of hypertonicity. This unwinding appears to occur at the level of the ground substance (matrix) of the connective tissue.
4. Use the Synchronizers™!

Application

1. Do not "use" the Tender Point. Pressure on these Tender Points will further stimulate the autonomic reflex arcs and will contribute to problems associated with existing hypertonicity.
2. Know where the Tender Point is situated if the treatment requires this knowledge. For example, position of the body part is occasionally relative to the location of the Tender Point.
3. Position the body, one-step-at-a-time, according to treatment directions. Maintain precisely the positions for at least one minute. Maintenance of the position for one minute will eliminate and/or decrease the hypertonicity of the contractile tissues.
4. Every technique should be continued beyond the one-minute duration in order to attain a De-Facilitated Fascial Release™. Maintain the position until the end of the release. The release is the tissue tension change and transformation, which can be palpated.
5. Use the Synchronizers™ for more effective and efficient results!

CHAPTER 5

ADVANCED STRAIN AND COUNTERSTRAIN FOR THE VISCERA

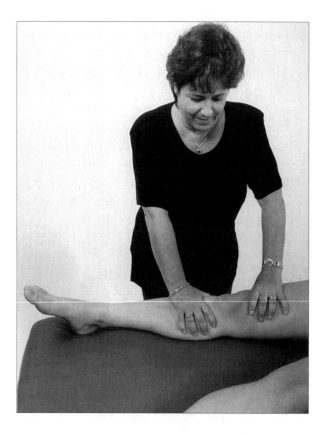

Org/UG2: Bladder

(Netter's plate # 341 - 348, 355, 357, 362)
(Bilateral)

TENDER POINT

On the inferior pubic ramus, at the medial border of the bone, 1 inch caudal from the inferior border of the pubic symphysis.

TREATMENT

- Supine.
- Abduct both hips 20 degrees.
- Internally rotate the ipsilateral hip 10 degrees.
- Extend the knee (straight leg).
- Internally rotate the tibia on the femur with one lb. of force.

GOAL

Alleviate the hypertonicity of the bladder muscle.

INTEGRATIVE MANUAL THERAPY™

This technique will decrease the hypertonicity of the bladder and can be used with the other Advanced Strain/Counterstrain techniques for the kidneys, ureter and urethra. Often incontinence is due to the muscle spasm of the bladder muscle. Edema of the legs can be associated with hypertonicity of the bladder. Muscle spasm of the bladder is common, often the result of prolonged pubic symphysis dysfunction. This technique can be performed with the Advanced Strain/Counterstrain Urogenital sequence.

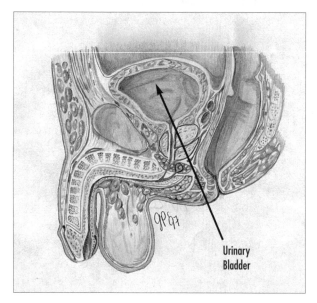

Urinary
Bladder

Org/UGF3: Cervix

(Netter's plate #341–352, 355)
(Bilateral)

TENDER POINT

There is no Tender Point for this musculature. The technique must be performed with the 'Mechanical Model.'

TREATMENT

- Supine.
- Flex both hips to 60 degrees.
- Knees are flexed to 50 degrees.
- Cross the legs, with the ipsilateral leg on top.
- Move both knees toward the ipsilateral side 20 degrees.

GOAL

To decrease hypertonicity of the cervix musculature.

INTEGRATIVE MANUAL THERAPY™

This technique will often affect pain, cramping, menstrual cramps, and other PMS symptomatology. This technique occasionally causes large changes in sitting pain and sitting tolerance. This technique can be performed with the Advanced Strain/Counterstrain Urogenital Sequence.

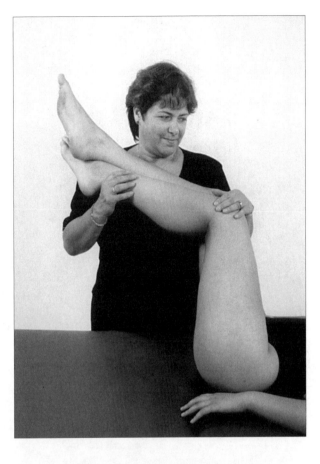

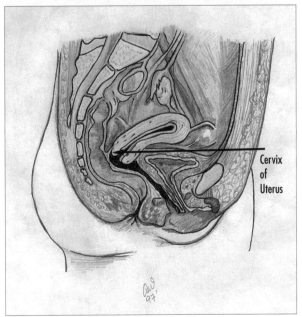

Cervix
of
Uterus

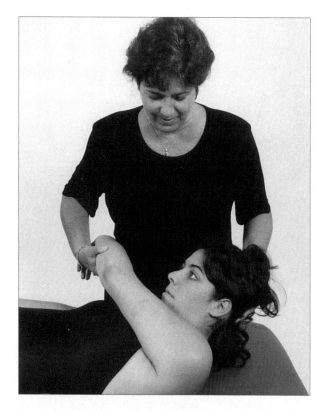

Org/HT1: Heart

(Netter's plate #182, 184, 194, 200, 202, 214)
(Unilateral)

TENDER POINT

1 inch left of the left 4th sternocostal joint and slightly inferior. (At the junction of the ventricles and atria which is approximately at the 4th rib.)

TREATMENT

- Supine.
- Neck flexion to the end of cervical range of motion.
- Neck sidebending to the right 10 degrees.
- Left shoulder in horizontal adduction to the end of range of motion.

GOAL

Release of the heart muscle.

INTEGRATIVE MANUAL THERAPY™

This technique is useful for all patients with chest tightness, and/or any rib cage symptomatology. There are no contra-indications to the use of this technique. There may be limitations of T3, T4, T5 mobility. There may be upper and/or mid-thoracic limitations of motion. There may be left shoulder girdle limitations of motion which are all indications for use of Org/HT1 Advanced Strain/Counterstrain technique.

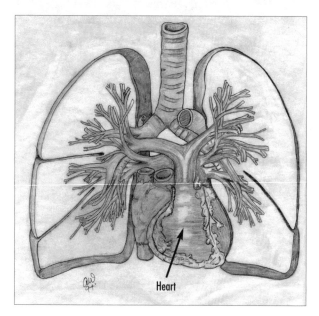

Heart

Org/LI1: Large Intestine 1

(Sigmoid colon)
(Netter's plate #267–269, 309, 310)
(Unilateral)

TENDER POINT

Posterior. Immediately above the iliac crest on the posterior surface of the colon on the left side.

TREATMENT

- Supine.
- Left hip flexion to 60 degrees.
- Knee straight.
- Left hip adduction to 10 degrees.

GOAL

Release of sigmoid colon.

INTEGRATIVE MANUAL THERAPY™

Limitations of lumbar extension, side bendings and rotations are good indications to use this technique. Abdominal cramps and pain on palpation of the abdomen is a reliable indication that this technique might be of assistance. Bowel dysfunction, for example constipation and/or diarrhea may be helped. There are no contra-indications to using this technique.

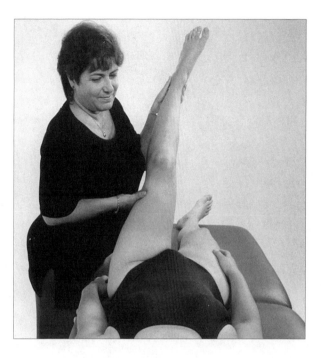

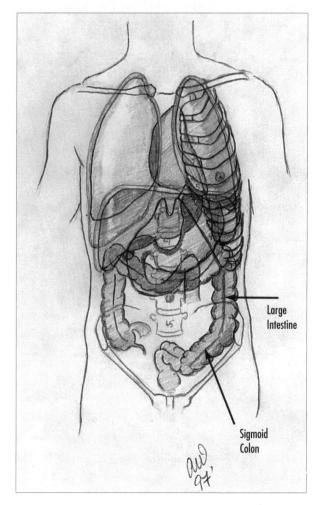

Large Intestine

Sigmoid Colon

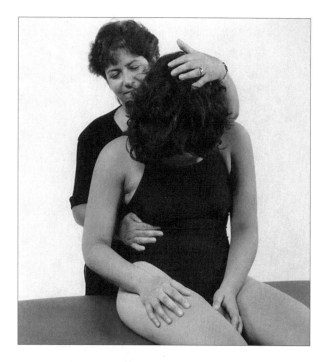

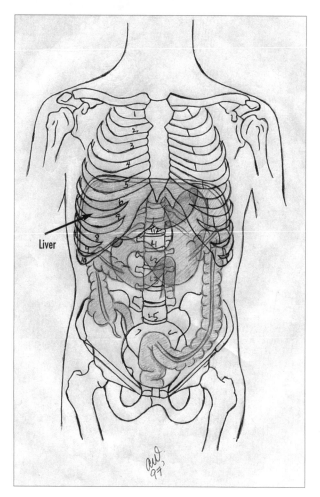

Liver

Org/LV1: Liver 1

(Netter's plate #184, 251, 269, 270, 302)
(Unilateral)

TENDER POINT

Upper edge of the falciform ligament of the liver. (At 8th costochondral cartilage on the right, 1½–1¾ inch lateral from midline.)

TREATMENT

- Sitting.
- Thoracic spine flexion to 60 degrees (To the upper edge of the liver).
- Thoracic spine rotation to the right to 30 degrees (for rotation of the "left" liver towards the "right" liver). (The "left" liver is on the left side of the falciform ligament of the liver. The "right" liver is on the right side of the falciform ligament of the liver.)
- Thoracic spine side bending 35 degrees to the left (For sidebending of the "left" liver from the "right" liver).

GOAL

Release of the liver.

INTEGRATIVE MANUAL THERAPY™

Contraction of liver tissue is common. Occasionally there will be a long-lasting effect of decreased rib cage pain on the right. Sometimes the limitations of right shoulder girdle movements will be reduced, or eliminated after performing this technique. Respiration will improve; rib excursion of the lower right ribs will increase. Changes in liver function will rarely occur.

Org/LU1: Lung 1

(Netter's plate #68, 182, 184–186)
(Bilateral)

TENDER POINT

Anterior/superior/medial tip of lung.

TREATMENT

- Sitting or Supine.
- Neck flexion to the end of cervical range of motion, without over-pressure.
- Ipsilateral shoulder into full horizontal adduction to the end of range of motion.

GOAL

Release of the lungs.

INTEGRATIVE MANUAL THERAPY™

This technique is extemely effective for increasing drainage at the thoracic inlet. The tension of the fibers attached to the dome of the lung will decrease. There will be increased joint mobility of the sternoclavicular joints, occasionally with large increases in shoulder girdle movements and significant improvements in cervicothoracic posture. There will always be increased cervical and upper thoracic ranges of motion. Lower neck movement will increase as pain in that region decreases.

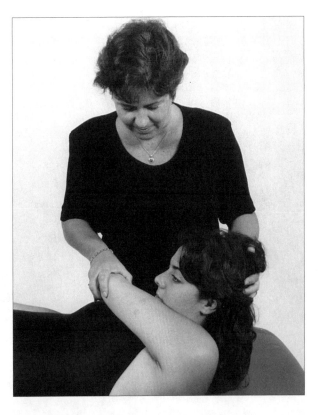

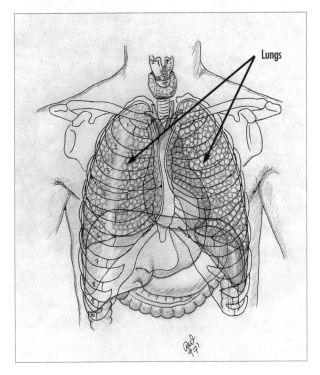

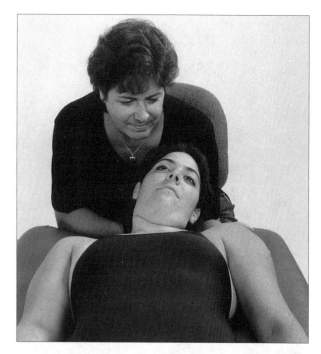

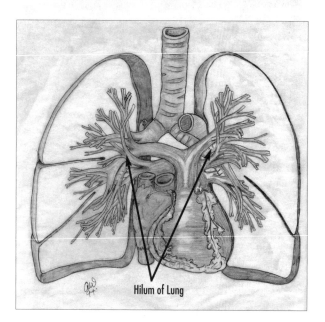

Hilum of Lung

Org/LU2: Hilum of Lung

(Netter's plate #184–187, 194, 218, 219)
(Bilateral)

TENDER POINT

2 cm lateral from the sternoclavicular joint, on the posterior surface of clavicle.

TREATMENT

- Supine.
- Cervical flexion 15 degrees.
- Cervical rotation to the ipsilateral side 10 degrees.
- Cervical side bending to the ipsilateral side 10 degrees.
- Protract the ipsilateral shoulder girdle one inch off the table (3 cm).

GOAL

Release of the smooth muscles of the hilum of the lung.

INTEGRATIVE MANUAL THERAPY™

This technique will alleviate: bronchial restrictions causing coughing, tension affecting respiration, choking, hiccuping, and allow chest expansion. Mediastinal tension will decrease. Because there is apparently an acid production area (which causes gout when stimulated inappropriately) at the junction of the aorta and the oesophagus, often there is a significant decrease in heartburn, reflux, and even the painful gout syndrome. This technique is good to use with all pulmonary and cardiovascular symptomotology. There are no contraindications with this technique.

Org/PN1: Pancreas 1

(Netter's plate #256, 257, 279, 280, 283, 294, 303)
(Unilateral)

TENDER POINT

Between the 5th and 6th rib on the left, 2 inches to the left of midline. (At the tail of the pancreas.)

TREATMENT

- Supine.
- Left leg abduction to 20 degrees.
- Trunk sidebending fully to the left.

GOAL

Release of the pancreas.

INTEGRATIVE MANUAL THERAPY™

This technique often results in significant improvements beyond expectation. The lower rib mobility will increase. There may be a decrease in indigestion, heartburn, and stomach pain. Lumbar movements will improve in all directions. Abdominal muscle spasms will decrease. There will be minimal improvement in pancreatic function.

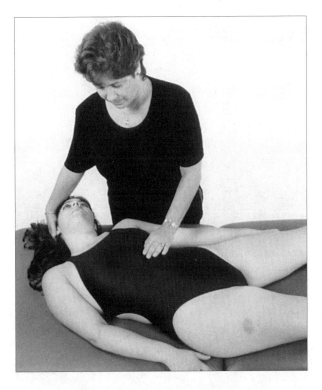

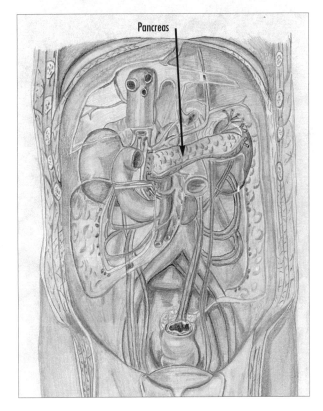

Pancreas

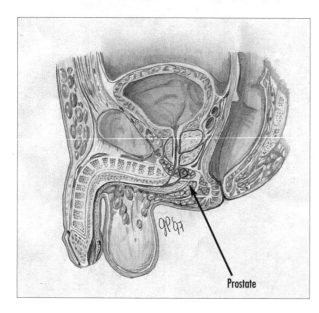

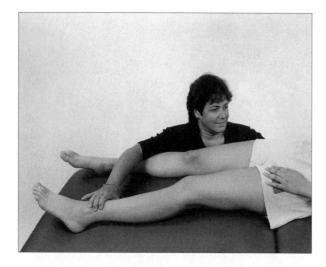

Prostate

Org/UGM1: Prostate 1

(Netter's plate #342, 362, 372, 378, 383, 391)
(Bilateral)

TENDER POINT

Tender point on the lower pubic bone on the posterior/inferior aspect of the bone, one inch lateral to the pubic symphysis.

TREATMENT

- Supine.
- Legs are abducted 15 degrees.
- Internal rotation of both legs.
- Low back is pushed anteriorly (force at waist level) with force of 10 lbs.

GOALS

Relaxed tone of the prostate which is required for normal hormone production.

INTEGRATIVE MANUAL THERAPY™

This technique may help the discomfort of prostatitis, which is common in men over 50 years old. Occasionally there will be a decrease in burning sensation experienced during urination. Often the client is experiencing indigestion, which may subside after this technique.

Org/SI1: Small Intestine 1

(Netter's plate #252, 286, 287, 296–301)
(Bilateral)

TENDER POINT

1 inch inferior to umbilicus, 2 inches obliquely inferior from this point at 45 degree angle from there.

TREATMENT

- Supine.
- Ipsilateral hip flexion to 60 degrees.
- Bilateral hip adduction. Legs are criss-crossed.
- Knees are straight.

GOAL

Release of small intestines.

INTEGRATIVE MANUAL THERAPY™

This technique is extremely helpful whenever there are abdominal cramps and discomfort. The effect will be short if there is an infectious process affecting the small intestines; in these cases relief will be provided for a short time (several hours). Otherwise, whenever palpation of the abdomen below the umbilicus is painful, this technique may be extremely effective. Always there will be an increase in hip extension and lumbar extension. Occasionally discogenic dysfunction will be helped by this technique. Sometimes there is a decrease in hip radicular pain after performing this technique.

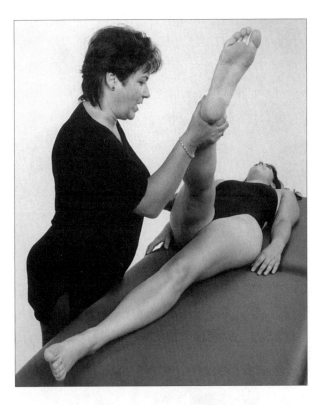

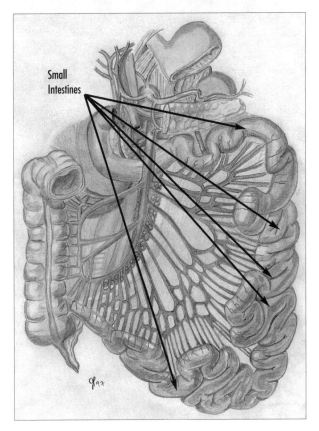

Small
Intestines

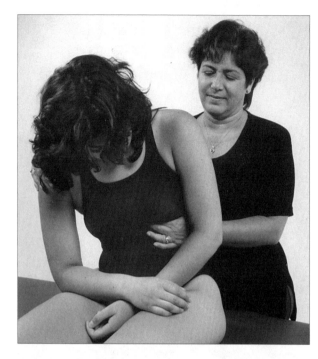

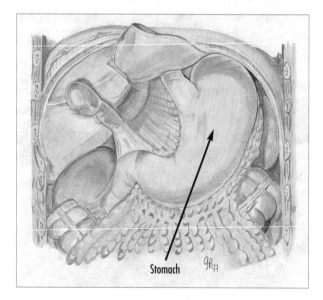

Stomach

Org/ST1: Stomach 1

(Netter's plate #220, 255, 256, 258, 307)
(Unilateral)

TENDER POINT

Tip of the xiphoid. 1/2 inch to 3/4 inch superior, slightly to the left. (At junction between the stomach and the cardiac sphincter of the stomach.)

TREATMENT

- Sitting.
- Thoracic spine flexion to 60 degrees (To the hiatus of the stomach).
- Thoracic spine rotation 35 degrees to the left towards the tender point.
- Thoracic spine sidebending to the right 20–30 degrees, away from the Tender Point.

GOAL

Release of the stomach.

INTEGRATIVE MANUAL THERAPY™

This technique, when used appropriately, will result in considerable decrease in stomach disorders and dysfunction. Often the acid-produced dysfunctions appear secondary to muscle spasm, and the client may be able to decrease medications for heartburn, indigestion, gastritis and even ulcers because of less pain. There is often a direct correlation to increased right shoulder girdle movement with decreased pain when this technique is performed.

Org/UGF1: Uterus 1

(Netter's plate #341–351, 372, 389)
(Bilateral)

TENDER POINT

Tender points on the anterior wall of the uterus at the junction of the uterus and fallopian tubes.

TREATMENT

- Abduct both straight legs to 15 degrees.
- Keep the legs straight.
- Bring legs straight up to the ceiling
- Internally rotate both lower extremities.

GOAL

Relaxed tone of the uterus, required for improved hormonal production.

INTEGRATIVE MANUAL THERAPY™

This technique will be appreciated by women who experience PMS. Often abdominal cramping is the result of spasm of the muscle of the uterus. This technique can be performed with the Advanced Strain/Counterstrain Urogenital sequence.

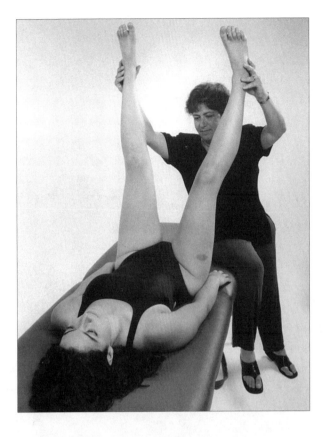

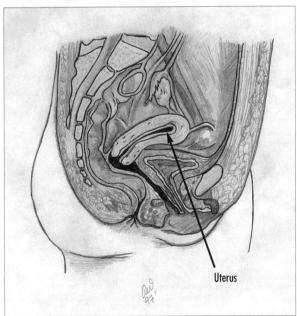

Uterus

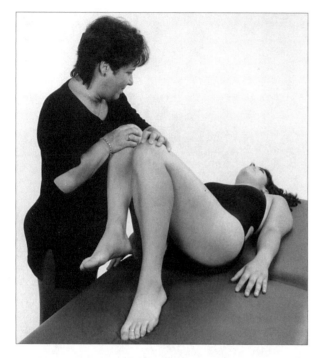

Org/UG1: Ureter

(Netter's plate #247, 248, 269, 325, 324)
(Bilateral)

TENDER POINT

1 inch above the superior medial border of the pubic symphysis, and 2 inches lateral.

TREATMENT

- Supine.
- Bend both hips and knees, with the feet on the table.
- The heels are together, approximately 6 inches inferior from the buttocks.
- Bring both knees together.
- Move both knees 7 inches lateral toward the ipsilateral side.
- The knees are 3 inches apart (separated).
- Then bring the ipsilateral knee toward the chest, so that the foot is 2 inches off the table.

GOAL

Elimination of hypertonicity of the ureter muscle.

INTEGRATIVE MANUAL THERAPY™

This technique will accompany treatment for kidney and blood pressure problems. Especially when there is a toxicity problem, for example with fibromyalgia-like syndromes, this technique will facilitate drainage of toxins. Often low back pain is the result of congestion of the ureters. This technique can be performed with the Advanced Strain/Counterstrain Urogenital sequence.

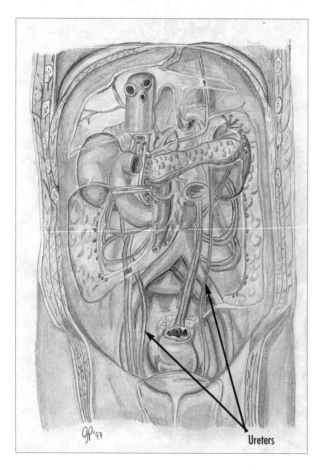

Ureters

Org/UG3: Urethra

(Netter's plate #341, 342, 363, 363)
(Bilateral)

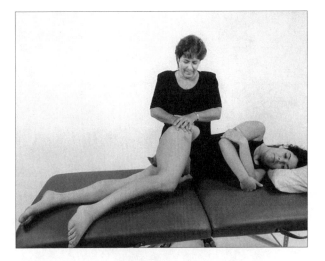

TENDER POINT

At the anterior, distal portion of the inferior pubic ramus, 1/2 inch lateral to the pubic symphysis.

TREATMENT

- Side lying on the side opposite the Tender Point (the contralateral side).
- Flex the bottom hip (contralateral) to 45 degrees.
- Flex the bottom knee (contralateral) to 45 degrees.
- Place a small towel roll between the hips, very close to the pubic symphysis.
- Flex the top hip (ipsilateral) to 60 degrees.
- Flex the top knee (ipsilateral) to 30 degrees.
- Compress lateral to medial (towards the floor) at the greater trochanter with one (1) lb. force.

GOAL

Eliminate spasm of the urethra musculature.

INTEGRATIVE MANUAL THERAPY™

This technique will facilitate urination. Often there will be decreased pain with urination. This technique occasionally causes large changes in sitting pain and sitting tolerance. This technique can be performed with the Advanced Strain / Counterstrain Kidney sequence.

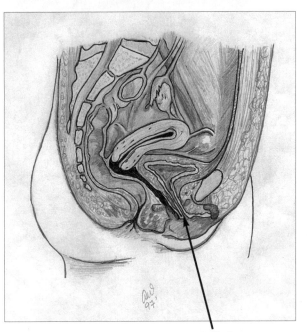

Urethra

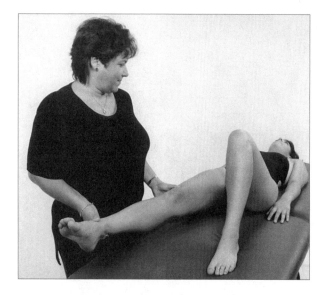

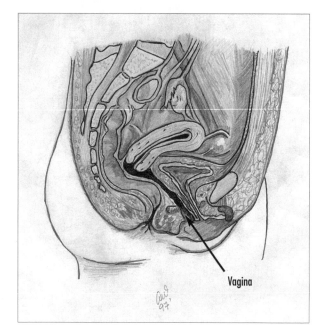

Vagina

Org/UGF2: Vagina
(Netter's plate #341–352, 355)
(Bilateral)

TENDER POINT

From the ASIS, one (1) inch medial and three (3) inches caudal.

TREATMENT

- Supine.
- Flex the opposite (contralateral) hip and knee, with the foot resting on the table.
- Abduct the ipsilateral hip to 30 degrees.
- Internally rotate the ipsilateral hip 10 degrees.
- Flex the ipsilateral hip 5 degrees with a straight leg.
- (Maintain knee extension.)

GOAL

To decrease hypertonicity of the vagina musculature.

INTEGRATIVE MANUAL THERAPY™

This technique will often affect pain, abdominal cramping, menstrual cramps, and other PMS symptomatology. Occasionally, persistent inflammatory conditions of the vagina will subside, and even disappear, after this technique. This technique can be performed with the Advanced Strain/Counterstrain Urogenital Sequence.

Org/UGM2: Vas Deferens

(Netter's plate #342, 365, 366)
(Bilateral)

TENDER POINT

There is no Tender Point for the musculature. The technique must be performed with the 'Mechanical Model.'

TREATMENT

- Supine.
- Separate both legs.
- Abduct both hips 30 degrees.
- Internally rotate the ipsilateral hip 10 degrees.
- Perform longitudinal distraction of the hip (pull at the hip, or elsewhere on the leg above the knee) with three (3) lbs. force.

GOAL

To decrease hypertonicity of the Vas Deferens musculature.

INTEGRATIVE MANUAL THERAPY™

This technique will often result in decreased pain during sitting, standing and ambulation activities. Often sexual activities will be less painful. This technique occasionally causes large changes in sitting pain and sitting tolerance. This technique can be performed with the Advanced Strain/Counterstrain Urogenital Sequence.

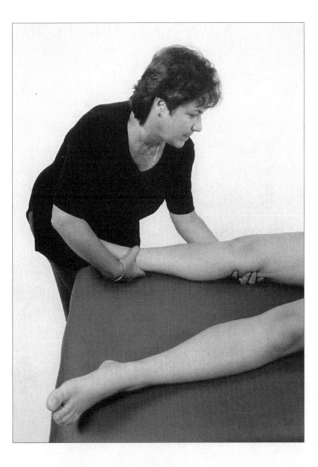

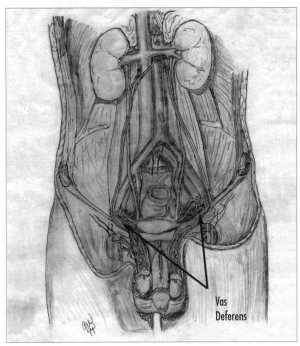

Vas
Deferens

ADVANCED STRAIN AND COUNTERSTRAIN FOR VISION

(Precaution: Please note if client is wearing contact lenses.)

The Ocular Muscles

Vis/1: Eye 1—Superior

(Netter's plate #76–81)

TENDER POINT

At the medial inner aspect of orbit.

TREATMENT

- Push eyeball towards nose, causing medial glide.
- Internally rotate eyeball.

GOAL

To look in a medial direction.

Vis/2: Eye 2—Inferior

(Netter's plate #76–81)

TENDER POINT

At the outer orbit, just caudal to pupil.

TREATMENT

- Push eyeball into caudal glide (inferior glide).
- Rotate posteriorly.

GOAL

To lower the eye.

Vis/3: Eye 3—Lateral

(Netter's plate #76–81)

TENDER POINT

At the outer orbit just above pupil.

TREATMENT

- Push eyeball into lateral glide.
- Externally rotate eyeball.

GOAL

To move eye to the outer peripheral field.

Vis/4: Eye 4—Inferomedial

(Netter's plate #76–81)

TENDER POINT

On the eyeball, at the inner and inferior corner of the eyeball.

TREATMENT

- Push eye towards nostrils in a direct glide(inferior/medial).

GOAL

To look down and in.

INTEGRATIVE MANUAL THERAPY™

Both eyes should ALWAYS be treated. Do not just treat one eye. It is possible to treat 2 eyes simultaneously, or first one eye, and next the second eye. The results of these techniques can be dramatic. Often there will be a defacilitation of the brain stem tissue and the sub-occipital tissue, leaving a remarkable improvement in upper cervical movement and decreased headaches and occipital tension. Vision may change, and there may be a need to change prescription of glasses. There may be a decrease in the tension of the tentorium cerebellum secondary to the defacilitation of the oculomotor, trochlear and abducens nerves (Cranial nerves 3, 4, 6).

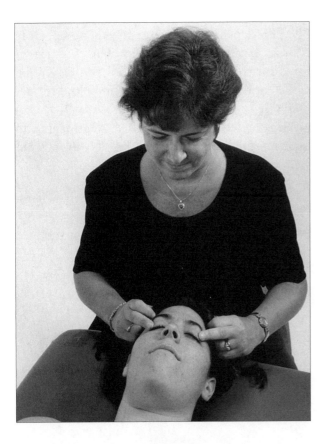
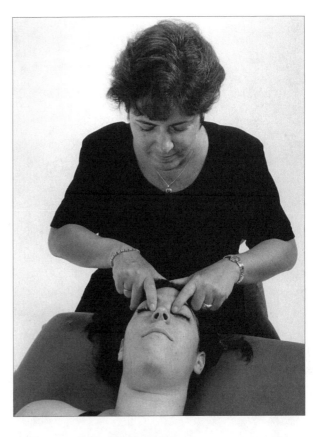
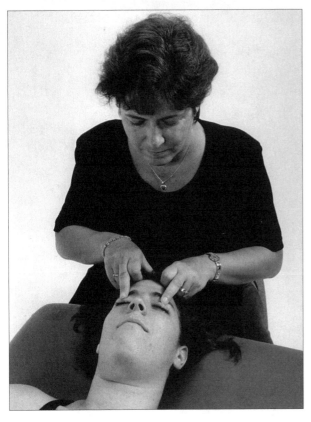
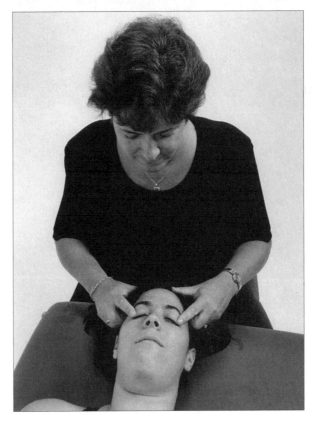

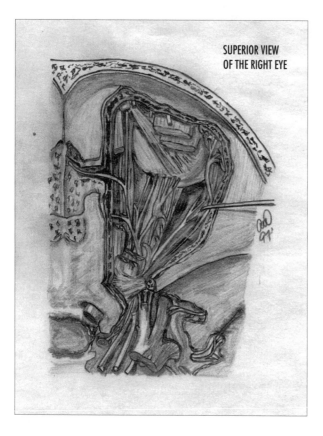

SUPERIOR VIEW
OF THE RIGHT EYE

NOTES: Do not press onto tender point. Only contact is required, with less than 1 gram of force for treatment. Hold for 1 minute. Will be sufficient to decrease hypertonicity. Hold for de-facilitated fascial release. Sequence 1-4, can progress bilateral, right and left treatments can be performed together. Hold E4 (#4) until brain stem defacilitation is complete.

CHAPTER 7

ADVANCED STRAIN AND COUNTERSTRAIN FOR AUDITORY FUNCTION

Aud/1: Tympanic Membrane
(Netter's plate #87–93)
(Bilateral)

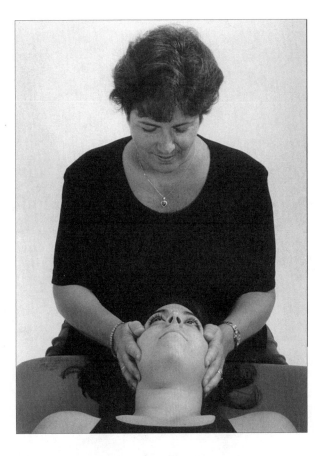

TENDER POINT

At the posterior aspect of the external auditory meatus, on the fibro-cartilaginous ear.

TREATMENT

- Supine.
- Therapist's hands cover both ears.
- Press both hands in a medial direction, squeezing with 5 grams of force.
- Head and neck are rotated 30 degrees towards the ipsilateral side.
- Maintain the 'squeeze' of 5 grams with both hands.
- Push on the fibrocartilagenous ear in a superior direction on the ipsilateral side of the Tender Point with 5 grams force.
- Press medial on the side of the Tender Point with an additional 5 grams of force.

GOAL

Release of the tympanic membrane.

INTEGRATIVE MANUAL THERAPY™

The practitioner using this technique on infants with ear infections will be "blessed" by the parents. The muscle spasm of the tympanic membrane is common, in all populations and all ages. The tympanic membrane is similar to a diaphragm, and contracts like a 'tent', the apex of the 'tent' at the medial aspect of the membrane. Hearing, equilibrium responses, ear symptoms will often be improved with this technique. Jaw pain and dysfunction will be surprisingly affected with this technique, because of the anatomic relationship between the tympanic membrane and the disc of the temporomandibular joint.

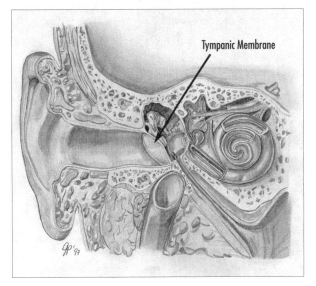

Tympanic Membrane

CHAPTER 8

ADVANCED STRAIN AND COUNTERSTRAIN FOR SPEECH AND SWALLOWING

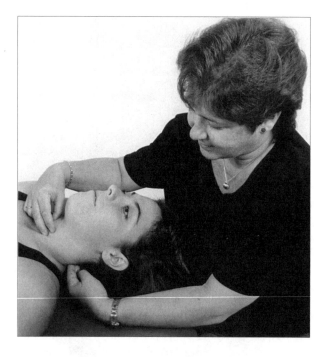

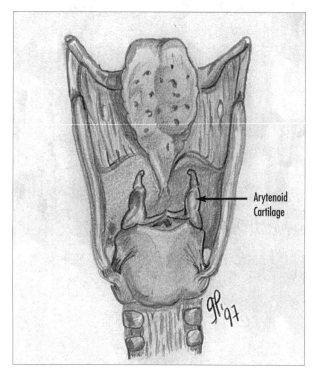

Arytenoid
Cartilage

Speech/1: Arytenoid Tendency to Adduct
(Netter's plate #71–73)
(Bilateral)

TENDER POINT

At the anterior-medial portion of the transverse process of C4.

TREATMENT

- Supine.
- Push the thyroid cartilage towards C4 transverse process on the ipsilateral side.
  (In cases of bilateral positive transverse processes, right side is generally treated first).
- Contact on the posterior lateral mass (in the cervical region). (The portion between the spinous processes and the transverse process is called the lateral mass.)
- Push C4 into an anterior shear on the ipsilateral side of the Tender Point.

GOAL

Allow arytenoid abduction. Correct arytenoid tendency to adduct.

INTEGRATIVE MANUAL THERAPY™

The vocal cords attach to the posterior aspect of the thyroid cartilage and at the arytenoid complexes ,anterior to the cervical spine at the level of C4 and C5. These muscles, the vocal cords, tend to adduct when they are in a state of protective muscle spasm. Speech and swallowing disorders can be alleviated with this technique. Often fascial restrictions remain, and require treatment with myofascial release after this technique. This technique can be performed after the myelohyoid is treated with Advanced Strain/Counterstrain.

Speech/2: Myelohyoid

(Netter's plate #57–67, 122)
(Bilateral)

TENDER POINT

Along the length of the insertion of the Myelohyoid, against the internal mandible at the
insertion, along the whole length of the
mandible.

TREATMENT

- Supine.
- Jaw is closed.
- Push the mandible in a lateral glide towards
  the ipsilateral side of the Tender Point with 5
  grams of force.
- Rotate the mandible to the ipsilateral side of
  Tender Point with 5 grams of force.
- Push the hyoid bone in a lateral glide
  towards the ipsilateral side of Tender Point
  with 5 grams force.
- Push the hyoid bone in a superior glide
  towards the ipsilateral side of Tender Point
  with 5 grams force.

GOAL

Relaxation of the tongue.

INTEGRATIVE MANUAL THERAPY™

This technique is effective for all hyoid and thyroid
cartilage restrictions. There will be improved function
of the tongue: proprioception, exteroception, coordination. The value of this technique for speech and temporomandibular problems cannot be over-emphasized.

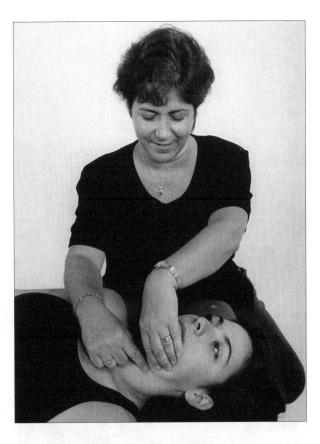

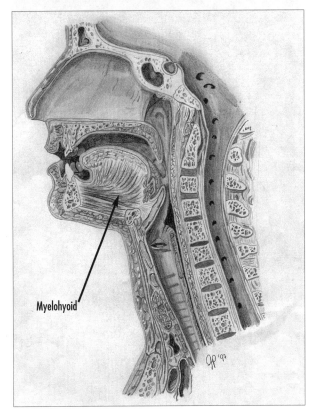

Myelohyoid

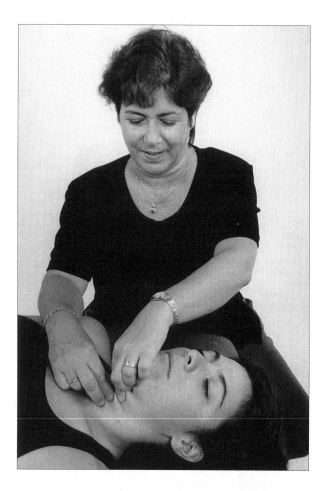

Speech/3: Thyroid cartilage elevation
(Netter's plate #57–67, 71–73)
(Bilateral)

TENDER POINT

At the anterior/superior/lateral corner of the thyroid cartilage.

TREATMENT

- Supine.
- Push the thyroid cartilage towards the Tender Point in a superior/lateral glide with 5 grams of force.
- Hyoid bone sidebending position towards the tender point.

GOAL

Elevation and depression of thyroid cartilage without crepitus.

INTEGRATIVE MANUAL THERAPY™

When the infrahyoid muscles are in a state of protective muscle spasm, the thyroid cartilage is held in elevation, which causes the sensation of a 'fist in the throat.' This technique can be used after the myelohoid technique. When the thyroid cartilage is held in a state of elevation, there is a tension on the thyroid gland, which can affect its function when this stress is chronic and severe. There are occasionally functional changes in thyroid gland function after performing this technique.

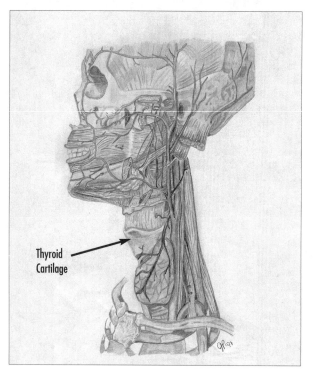

Thyroid
Cartilage

Speech/4: Vocal Cords

(Netter's plate #57–67, 71–73)
(Bilateral)

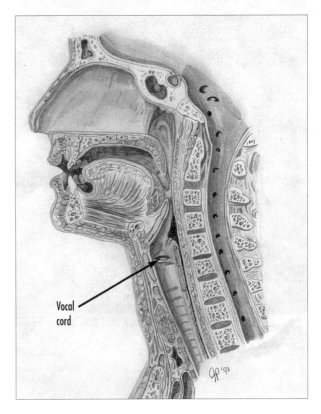

TENDER POINT

Tender Point is on the vocal cords, at their right and left insertion at the posterior body of the thyroid cartilage.

TREATMENT

- Supine.
- Adduct both of the walls of the thyroid cartilage.
- Perform a 3-planar articular fascial release (Weiselfish-Giammatteo, Myofascial Release). The articulation is the fascial interface of the right and left walls of the thyroid cartilage.

GOAL

Improved vocal cord tolerance.

INTEGRATIVE MANUAL THERAPY™

Protective muscle spasm of the vocal cords is a common occurrence, found often in clients with craniofacial pain, craniocervical and craniomandibular disorders. This dysfunction is a unique misfortune for those who sing and/or speak for a living!

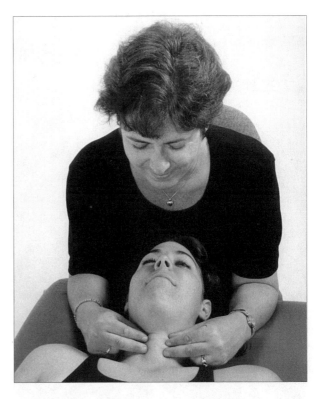

Vocal cord

CHAPTER 9

ADVANCED STRAIN AND COUNTERSTRAIN FOR THE DIAPHRAGM SYSTEM

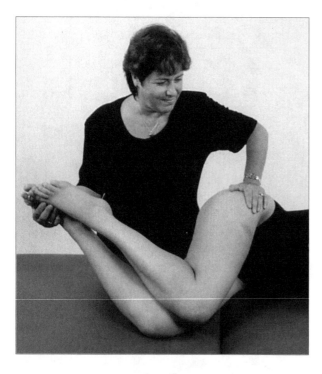

Diaph/1: Pelvic Diaphragm

(Netter's plate #337–342, 367, 368)
(Bilateral)

TENDER POINT

At the sacrococcygeal ligament, next to the ischial tuberosity.

TREATMENT

- Side lying.
- Lie on the contralateral side.
- Hips bilaterally flexed to 70 degrees.
- Knees bilaterally flexed to 70 degrees.
- Lift both feet up towards the ceiling, until the feet are 6 inches off the table.
- Push on the ilium, from 2 inches inferior from the iliac crest, mid-axillary line. Push with 3 lbs of force.

GOAL

Release the hypertonicity of the pelvic floor musculature.

INTEGRATIVE MANUAL THERAPY™

This technique can be performed prior to myofascial release of the pelvic diaphragm, and should be performed bilateral. This technique can be used together with the other three (3) diaphragm techniques for the respiratory abdominal diaphragm, the thoracic inlet and the cranial diaphragm. The pelvic soft tissue is almost always contracted in a state of spasm, especially because of the incidence of sacroiliac biomechanical dysfunction. This technique can be used during pregnancy, during labor to facilitate delivery, and immediately after delivery to promote healing of the pelvic floor. If there are stitches, because of episiotomy, or

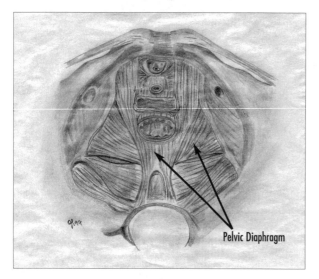

Pelvic Diaphragm

tearing of the pelvic floor during delivery, this technique can be repeated several times during the first week or two after childbirth for improved function. Whenever there is swelling of the legs, whether at an ankle after a sprain, or total leg edema, this technique may be invaluable. There are no precautions for this technique.

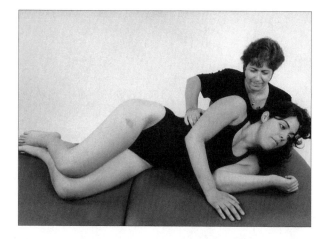

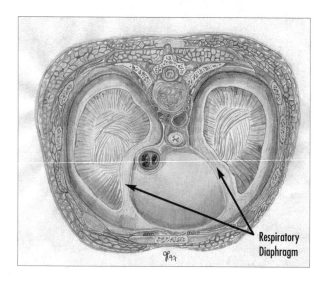

Respiratory
Diaphragm

Diaph/2: Respiratory Abdominal Diaphragm
(Netter's plate #180, 181, 183, 218, 219)
(Bilateral)

TENDER POINT

Bilateral, under the 10th rib, about 5 inches lateral from sternum.

TREATMENT

- Lie on the contralateral side.
- Hips are flexed to 50 degrees.
- Knees are fully flexed.
- Cervical sidebending to the end of range of motion without overpressure (coronal plane).
- Press on lower lateral rib cage towards the floor (to opposite side).

GOAL

Improve breathing.

INTEGRATIVE MANUAL THERAPY™

This technique will eliminate protective muscle spasm of the respiratory abdominal diaphragm, and is excellent to perform for all pulmonary, cardiac, and spinal patients. Because all four (4) diaphragms function as a complex, it is best to treat all four (4) diaphragms (the pelvic diaphragm, the thoracic inlet, the cranial diaphragm). After treatment with Advanced Strain/Counterstrain techniques for the diaphragm/s, myofascial release for the transverse fascial restrictions can be performed with increased effectivity. There are no precautions for this technique.

Diaph/3: Thoracic Inlet

(Netter's plate #168, 169, 175, 219)
(Bilateral)

TENDER POINT

Middle of supraspinous fossa, 1 inch medial from the medial aspect of the acromioclavicular joint, mid-way between clavicle and spine of scapula.

TREATMENT

- Side lying on the contra-lateral side.
- Use a pillow so the head and neck are mid-line (no cervical side-bending).
- Ipsilateral shoulder abduction to 70 degrees.
- Ipsilateral shoulder girdle depression, inferior with 3 lbs. of force.

GOAL

Release of hypertonicity of thoracic inlet muscles.

INTEGRATIVE MANUAL THERAPY™

This technique can be used prior to all cranial therapy. The CSF production will be enhanced whenever cranial mobilization is performed, and both the craniocervical region as well as the thoracic inlet must be open for drainage. This technique can be used prior to myofascial release of the diaphragms. All of the diaphragms function together as a unit. One of the four diaphragms (pelvic, respiratory abdominal, thoracic inlet, and cranial) in a state of dysfunction will affect the status of all of the other diaphragms. The lymph terminus drains into the thoracic inlet; the terminus can be located in the immediate vicinity where the jugular vein penetrates the thoracic inlet. Lymphatic drainage can be uniquely affected by thoracic inlet diaphragm spasm. The lymphatic drainage of both legs, and the abdomen drain into the cistern chyle, and from there into the thoracic duct. The left arm, the left neck and head and face all drain together, with the legs and the abdomen into the left thoracic inlet, into the vena cava and into

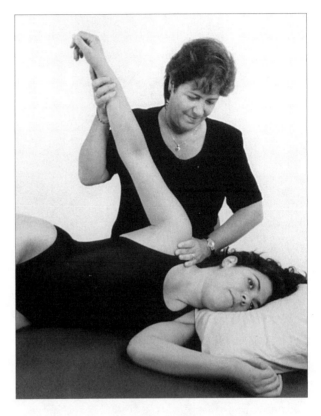

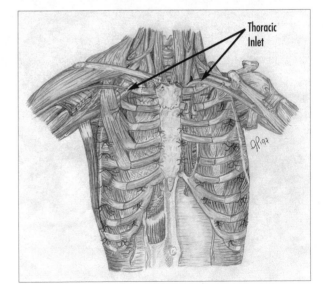

Thoracic Inlet

the heart. Through the right thoracic inlet there is lymphatic drainage only of the lungs and chest, right arm and head and face. Therefore, 75% of lymphatic drainage flows via the left thoracic inlet. When the left thoracic inlet is in a state of hypertonicity, there is congestion, and toxins with excess fluid remain in the interstitium, causing swelling and myofascial dysfunction. Observe the legs and abdomen and left upper quadrant: when edematous and painful to palpation, this technique will result in remarkable changes, including decreased pain, swelling and spasm. All head and neck and upper quadrant patients will respond well to this technique. This technique can be used together with the Advanced Strain /Counterstrain techniques for the other three diaphragms. Typically this technique, and the other diaphragm techniques, will respond best with bilateral treatment. There are no precautions for this technique.

Diaph/4: Subclavius

(Netter's plate #395, 404)
(Bilateral)

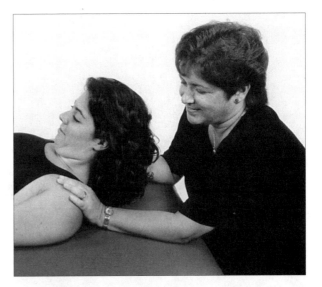

TENDER POINT

At middle of the subclavius muscle, on the insertion at the clavicle, on the inferior bony surface.

TREATMENT

- Supine.
- Lift head and neck into full cervical flexion without over pressure.
- Compress the ipsilateral shoulder girdle inferior (shoulder girdle depression) with hand over superior aspect of shoulder girdle.

GOAL

Open the Costoclavicular joint space.

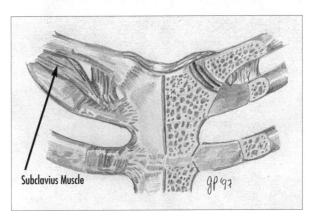

Subclavius Muscle

INTEGRATIVE MANUAL THERAPY™

This technique is excellent to add to the protocol for thoracic outlet syndrome. When there is compression of the brachial plexus in the costoclavicular joint space, this technique can be used with the following protocol to decompress clavicle from the first rib: (a) Jones anterior first thoracic technique; Jones anterior C7 and C8 techniques: the sternoclavicular joint will open; (b) Jones anterior and posterior acromioclavicular techniques: the acromioclavicular joint will open; (c) Jones elevated first rib technique; Jones lateral cervical techniques for the scalenes: the first rib will drop from its elevated position; (d) Subclavius Advanced Strain/Counterstrain technique will eliminate the compression on the subclavian artery and there should be a restoration of improved circulation.

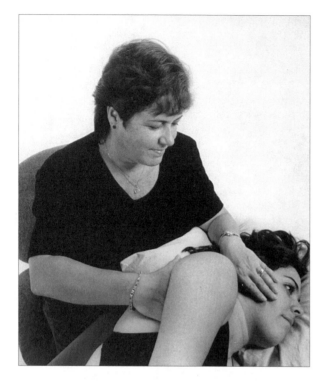

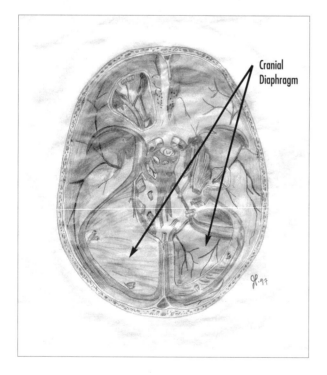

Cranial
Diaphragm

Diaph/5: Cranial Diaphragm

(Netter's plate #97, 98, 100)
(Bilateral)
(The cranial diaphragm is the combined tentorium cerebellum and foramen magnum contractile tissues.)

TENDER POINT

Just caudal to the fibrocartilagenous ear, directly aligned with the meatus, on the anterior aspect of the mastoid.

TREATMENT

- Sidelying on the contra-lateral.
- Place palm of hand over ear (meatus) with fingers also covering the temporal bone superior to the meatus.
- Press on the ipsilateral temporal and meatus lateral to medial with 5 grams of force.
- Place a hand in axilla on the ipsilateral side.
- Push from the inferior aspect of axilla up towards the meatus of the ear.

GOAL

Release the hypertonicity of the cranial diaphragm.

INTEGRATIVE MANUAL THERAPY™

This remarkable technique is used for specific problems, and also just to improve diaphragm function. All four diaphragms (pelvic, respiratory abdominal, thoracic inlet and cranial) function as a unit. When one diaphragm is in a state of dysfunction, all the other diaphragms will be in some degree of hypertonicity. This technique can be performed prior to using cranial therapy. Often there is a change in vision, because the tentorium cerebellum is no longer compressing on the cranial nerves which innervate the ocular muscles (oculomotor, trochlear, abducens) that pass through the tentorium. Ear pain, tinnitus, ear stuffiness, hearing, equilibrium may all improve with this technique. With seizure disorders there is occasionally a significant improvement. All head, face and neck pain patients can benefit from this technique. There will often be excellent improvements when this technique is used during acute phase of neurologic disorders, because there will be improved drainage of CSF when the cranial diaphragm is not in spasm. There are no precautions for this technique.

CHAPTER 10

ADVANCED STRAIN AND COUNTERSTRAIN FOR ELEMENTAL CIRCULATORY VESSELS

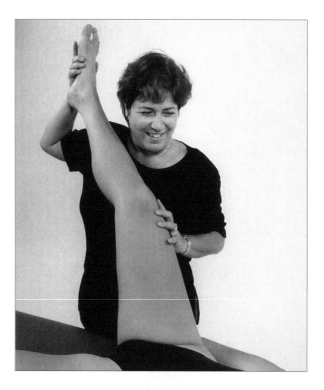

Circ/1: Circulatory Vessels of the Lower Extremities

(Netter's plate #481, 487, 489)
(Bilateral)

TENDER POINT

On the inner, upper thigh, medial at mid-line, 4 inches below the pubic bone.

TREATMENT

- Supine.
- Hip flexion to 90 degrees.
- Hip abduction to 30 degrees.
- Hip externally rotate to 25 degrees.
- Knee is in full extension (not locked).
- Ankle plantar flexion to 20 degrees.
- Foot is pronated: hind foot, mid-foot, fore-foot to 15 degrees.

GOAL

Release of the smooth muscles of the lower extremities blood vessels.

INTEGRATIVE MANUAL THERAPY™

This technique will affect circulation of the leg, including arterial flow, venous return and lymphatic drainage. This will not eliminate severe hypertonicity of arteries, veins or lymph. For those severe circumstances, use the specific techniques, rather than this general technique. Yet this technique can precede specific leg circulatory Advanced Strain and Counterstrain techniques in order to minimize treatment reactions. This technique is excellent for soft tissue dysfunction, including myofascial dysfunction, scar tissue, protective muscle spasm, and other less circulatory-specific problems.

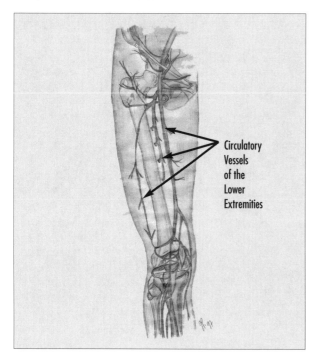

Circulatory Vessels of the Lower Extremities

Circ/2: Circulatory Vessels of the Upper Extremities

(Netter's plate #446)
(Bilateral)

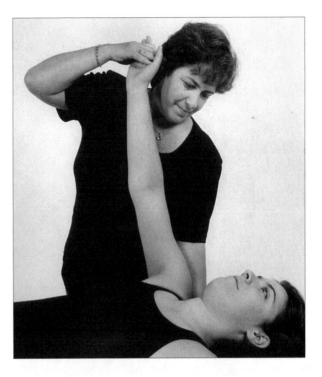

TENDER POINT

At the axilla, under the pectoralis major, on the axilla crease line.

TREATMENT

- Supine.
- Place a hand posterior to the neck.
- Push C7 and T1 into a lateral glide towards the ipsilateral side with 5 grams of force.
- Shoulder girdle is maximally protracted, without over pressure.
- Shoulder flexion to 90 degrees.
- Shoulder abduction 40 degrees.
- Shoulder internal rotation to 20 degrees.
- Elbow is extended (not locked).
- Forearm is supinated fully (not locked).
- Wrist extension to 20 degrees.
- Wrist radial deviation to 10 degrees.
- Thumb abducted to 20 degrees.
- Thumbs extended to 10 degrees.
- Finger joints (all) with full extension (not locked).

GOAL

Release of the smooth muscles of the upper extremities blood vessels.

INTEGRATIVE MANUAL THERAPY™

This technique will result in improved circulation of the arm. Arterial flow, venous return, and lymphatic drainage will all be affected. This technique can be utilized for the following purposes: to decrease pain from soft tissue dysfunction; to improve circulation secondary to soft tissue dysfunction; to decrease edema secondary to soft tissue dysfunction. This technique will be less effective for significant circulatory dysfunction, but can be used to precede techniques which are artery, vein and lymph specific, to eliminate any treatment reactions. Excellent results with fascial dysfunction are attained with this technique.

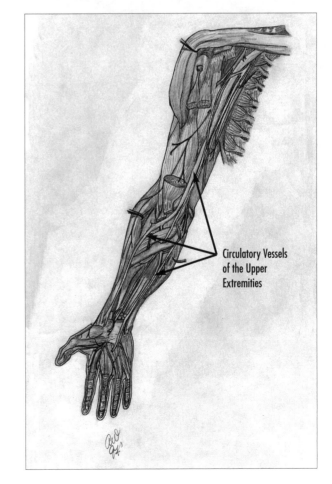

Circulatory Vessels of the Upper Extremities

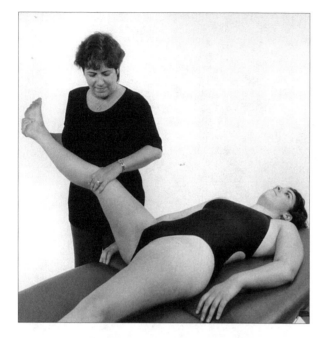

Circ/3: Circulatory Vessels of the Abdomen
(Netter's plate #238, 247, 248, 282–287)
(Bilateral)

TENDER POINT

1 inch inferior and 2 inches lateral to the umbilicus.

TREATMENT

- Supine.
- Hip flexion on the ipsilateral side to 120 degrees.
- Hip full abduction, without over pressure.
- Hip full external rotation with 1 lb of force.
- Knee is in full extension (not locked).
- Ankle plantar flexion to 20 degrees.
- Foot is supinated: hind-foot, mid-foot, fore-foot to 10 degrees.

GOAL

Release of the smooth muscles of the abdominal blood vessels.

INTEGRATIVE MANUAL THERAPY™

This technique is excellent for general loss of circulation and edema affecting the abdominal cavity. Good results are often attained with cramps. Specific techniques of Advanced Strain and Counterstrain will be required for more significant circulatory-specific problems, but this technique is good to precede the specific techniques in order to decrease treatment reactions.

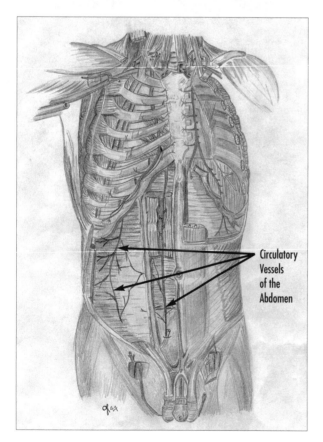

Circulatory Vessels of the Abdomen

Circ/4: Circulatory Vessels of the Chest Cavity
(Netter's plate #175, 176, 179, 238)

TENDER POINT

3 inches inferior to nipple line (align soft tissue). Usually on the intracostal soft tissue between ribs 6 and 7.

TREATMENT

- Supine.
- Upper body flexion. Flex down the spinal kinetic chain to the level of T6.
- Ipsilateral shoulder flexion to 90 degrees.
- Ipsilateral shoulder horizontal adduction with over pressure of 1 lb. force.
- Elbow extension (not locked).

GOAL

Release of the smooth muscles of the chest blood vessels.

INTEGRATIVE MANUAL THERAPY™

This technique will facilitate improved circulation within the chest cavity. Decreased effects from intra-thoracic edema will result in improved rib excursion and respiration. For more severe respiratory problems, including asthma, COPD, emphysema, atelectasis, this technique can precede the more specific techniques, in order to decrease treatment reactions. For example, this technique can be used (bilateral) prior to the Advanced Strain and Counterstrain techniques for the coronary arteries. Use for all thoracic, neck and rib cage clients. There are no contra-indications.

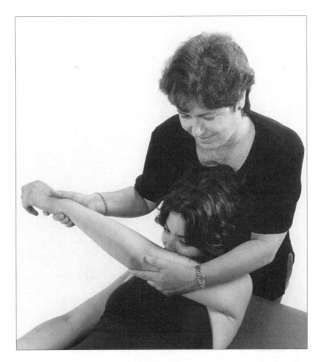

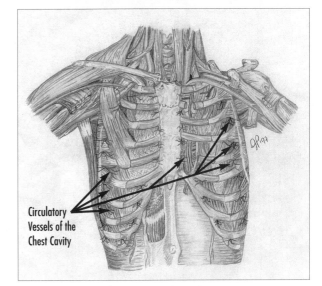

Circulatory Vessels of the Chest Cavity

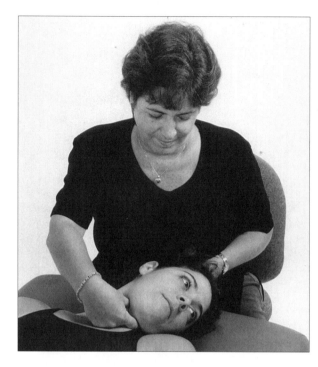

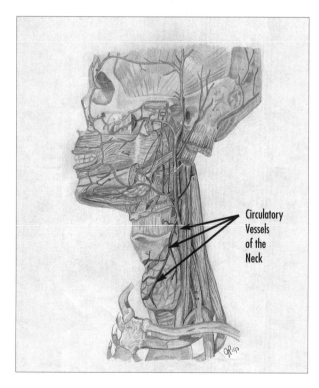

Circulatory
Vessels
of the
Neck

Circ/5: Circulatory Vessels of the Neck
(Netter's plate #63)
(Bilateral)

TENDER POINT

Lateral neck, on the soft tissue at C2, just anterior to mid-axillary line.

TREATMENT

- Supine.
- Neck rotation to the end of range to the ipsilateral side, without over pressure.
- Neck sidebending to the ipsilateral side to the end of range, without over pressure.
- Hyoid bone is grasped between the index finger and thumb.
- Push the hyoid bone into lateral glide toward the Tender Point, towards the ipsilateral side, without over pressure.

GOAL

Release of the smooth muscles of the neck blood vessels.

INTEGRATIVE MANUAL THERAPY™

The therapist will occasionally be surprised with the results of this technique. Because the body protects arteries and veins, often when there is mild tension of the circulatory vessels, the neck will deviate towards the side of the problem, causing other secondary cervical problems. When the Advanced Strain and Counterstrain is performed, the neck may have markedly increased ranges of motion, without any residual problems remaining at the cervical region. Use for all head, face and neck problems with all patients. There are no contraindications.

Circ/6: Circulatory Vessels of the Cranial Vault

(Netter's plate #95)
(Bilateral)

TENDER POINT

Lift up the ear lobe. The Tender Point is on the fibrocartilaginous ear, posterior aspect, 1 cm superior from inferior (distal) edge of ear lobe. From this point, go posterior 1 inch.

TREATMENT

- Supine.
- Grasp the ipsilateral fibrocartilagenous ear.
- Glide the ipsilateral fibrocartilagenous ear in a posterior direction towards the Tender Point.

GOAL

Release of the smooth muscles of the cranial vault blood vessels.

INTEGRATIVE MANUAL THERAPY™

This technique will not be effective for migraine patients with significant spasm of the arteries, veins, and lymph within the cranial vault. But this technique is excellent used prior to other specific techniques, to reduce treatment reactions. For example, this technique can be used before the Advanced Strain and Counterstrain for the cerebral arteries. Although there are no contraindications for this technique, PRECEDE THIS TECHNIQUE WITH THE ADVANCED STRAIN AND COUNTERSTRAIN TECHNIQUES FOR THE DIAPHRAGMS: (a) PELVIC DIAPHRAGM, (b) RESPIRATORY ABDOMINAL DIAPHRAGM, (c) THORACIC INLET DIAPHRAGM, AND (d) CRANIAL DIAPHRAGM. Then there will not be problems of congestion and poor drainage of CSF from the cranial vault through the thoracic inlet.

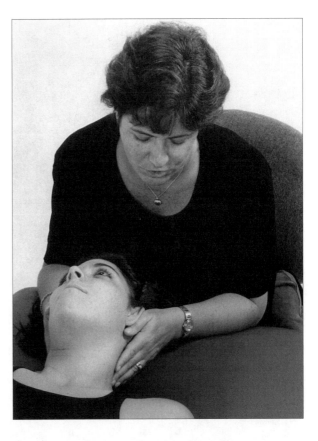

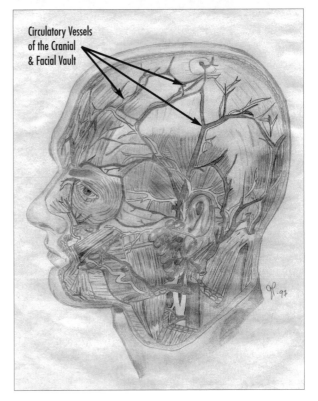

Circulatory Vessels of the Cranial & Facial Vault

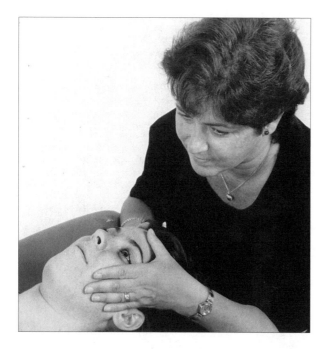

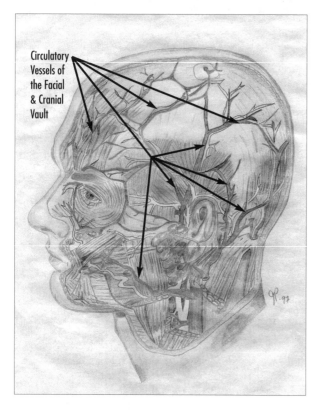

Circulatory Vessels of the Facial & Cranial Vault

Circ/7: Circulatory Vessels of the Facial Vault
(Netter's plate #17)
(Bilateral)

TENDER POINT

Masseter muscle, upper border, at the anterior insertion of the muscle at the bone.

TREATMENT

- Supine.
- Grasp masseter muscle and compress the muscle medial.
- Push the masseter muscle medial towards the ipsilateral zygoma, towards the Tender Point.

GOAL

Release of the smooth muscles of the facial vault blood vessels.

INTEGRATIVE MANUAL THERAPY™

This technique is good for all cranio-facial-mandibular pain and dysfunction. For example, mild temporalis arteritis will be affected by this technique, which is common in patients with temporomandibular joint disorders. Aging often affects the soft tissues of the face, and causes poor venous return, congestion, and lymph back-up. Overall, an excellent technique without any contra-indications. Good for facial scarring after surgery and trauma.

CHAPTER 11

ADVANCED STRAIN AND COUNTERSTRAIN FOR THE MUSCLES OF LYMPHATIC VESSELS

Lymph/1: Lower Extremities Lymphatic Vessels

(Netter's plate #249, 514)
(Bilateral)

TENDER POINT

At the groin; on the inferior pubic ramus, not on the tendon of the adductor magnus, but an inch medial from the tendon insertion.

TREATMENT

- Supine.
- Hip and knee flexion of the contralateral side; the foot rests on the bed.
- Hip flexion of the ipsilateral side 100 degrees on the ipsilateral side.
- Hip abduction of the ipsilateral 20 degrees on the ipsilateral side.
- Hip internal rotation 45 degrees on the ipsilateral side.
- Knee flexion of the ipsilateral side 100 degrees on the ipsilateral side.
- Ankle plantar flexion 10 degrees.
- Foot pronation (hind-foot, mid- foot, fore-foot) 20 degrees.

GOAL

Release of the smooth muscles of the lymphatic vessels of the lower extremities.

INTEGRATIVE MANUAL THERAPY™

This technique will restore lymphatic drainage in many clients who have mild to severe edema, which is a surprise. In other words, the effects of this technique are greater than would be anticipated. Excellent results may occur with pain, edema, scarring, burns, myofascial dysfunction, and all types of fibromyalgia-like presentations. Good results with acute and chronic burns.

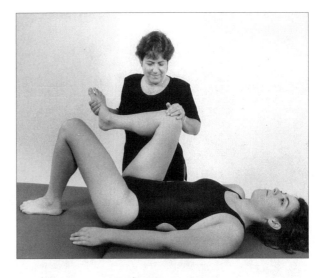

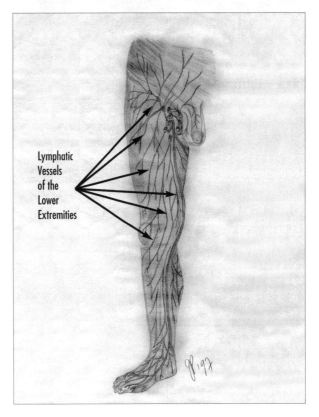

Lymphatic Vessels of the Lower Extremities

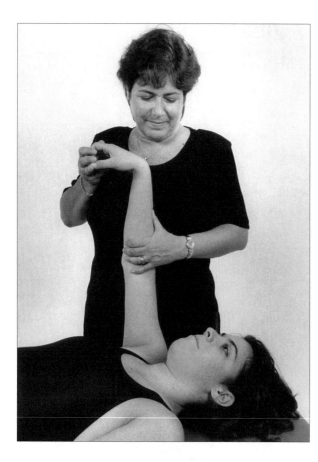

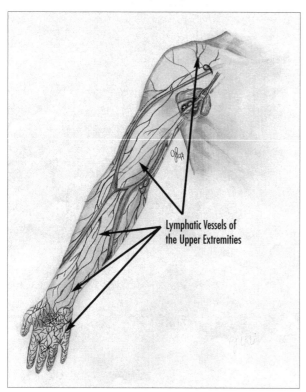

Lymphatic Vessels of
the Upper Extremities

Lymph/2: Upper Extremities Lymphatic Vessels
(Netter's plate #169, 456)
(Bilateral)

TENDER POINT

At the axilla, at the lateral border of the neck of humerus, level of axilla crease, on the bone.

TREATMENT

- Supine.
- Flexion of the shoulder to 90 degrees.
- No rotation of shoulder.
- Abduction of the shoulder to 25 degrees.
- Flexion of the elbow to 5 degrees.
- Pronation of the forearm to 70 degrees.
- Wrist flexion to 30 degrees.
- Wrist ulnar deviation to 25 degrees.
- Thumb flexion to 25 degrees.
- Thumb abduction to 20 degrees.
- Thumb opposition (from this starting place bring thumb towards 5th digit) 35 degrees.
- Finger flexion of all of the metacarpalphalangeal joints 30 degrees.
- Finger flexion of all of the proximal interphalangeal joints 20 degrees.
- Finger flexion of all of the distal interphalangeal joints 20 degrees.

GOAL

Release of the smooth muscles of the lymphatic vessels of the upper extremities.

INTEGRATIVE MANUAL THERAPY™

This general Advanced Strain and Counterstrain technique is good for all clients with edema, myofascial dysfunction, and pain of the upper quadrant. There will be a generalized effect of improved lymphatic drainage from the upper extremity into the lymph terminus at the thoracic inlet. Scarring post surgery and/or trauma is beneficially affected by this technique. Interestingly, even when the lymph nodes are removed or scarred from radiation, there is an extremely good effect of improved lymphatic drainage with this technique. The 'watershed' system of moving the lymph load from the affected side towards the non-affected side for drainage appears to be stimulated when hypertonicity of the lymphatic vessel musculature is decreased with this technique. Anticipate good results with acute and chronic burns.

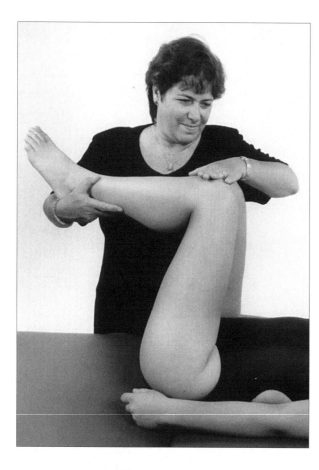

Lymph/3: Abdomen Lymphatic Vessels
(Netter's plate #249, 299, 300–303, 325)
(Bilateral)

TENDER POINT

Lower abdominal quadrant, 1 inch medial from the ASIS, 2 inches inferior from that point (in the inguinal tunnel).

TREATMENT

- Supine.
- Flex bilateral hips to 90 degrees.
- Flexion of both knees to 90 degrees.
- Posterior compression force from anterior aspect of knees towards the tender point of ipsilateral side.

GOAL

Release of the smooth muscles of the lymphatic vessels of the lower extremities.

INTEGRATIVE MANUAL THERAPY™

This technique will affect edema , cramps , myofascial dysfunction and pain within the abdominal cavity. The best way to utilize this technique is to use it in conjunction with Visceral Manipulation (Barral). It has increased effectivity when used with Jones Anterior Lumbar Strain and Counterstrain techniques.

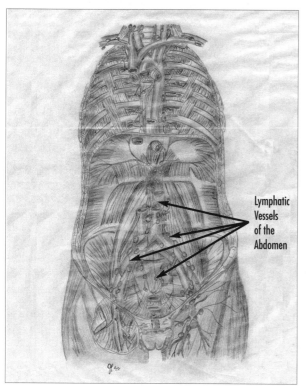

Lymphatic Vessels of the Abdomen

Lymph/4: Chest Cavity Lymphatic Vessels
(Netter's plate #197)
(Bilateral)

TENDER POINT

On the 4th rib, just medial to the angle of the rib, on the superior surface of the rib.

TREATMENT

- Supine.
- Flexion of the neck to the end of range without over pressure.
- Shoulder girdle protraction of the ipsilateral shoulder girdle with 1 lb. force of over pressure.
- Compression of the upper rib cage of the ipsilateral side towards the tender point on the posterior aspect of the rib.

GOAL

Release of the smooth muscles of the lymphatic vessels of the chest cavity.

INTEGRATIVE MANUAL THERAPY™

There is surprising benefit with this technique, beyond anticipated outcomes. There will be an excellent reduction in intra-thoracic swelling with all kinds of pulmonary disorders. After direct trauma, for example with seat belt injury in motor vehicle accidents, this technique can be performed immediately, so that intra-thoracic bleeding and swelling may be addressed for enhanced lymphatic drainage. There is no contra-indication with this technique. It can be used for all cardio-vascular and cardiopulmonary patients, before and/or after (immediately post-operation) any surgery.

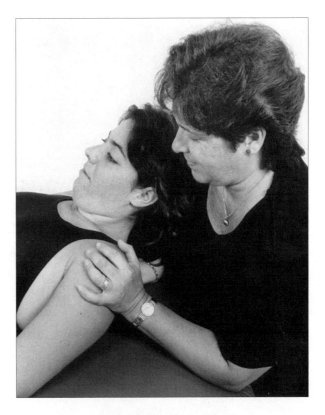

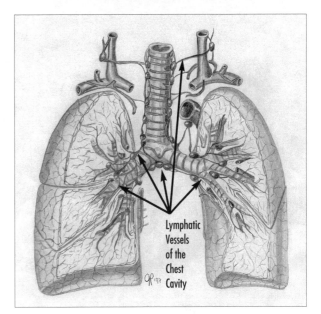

Lymphatic Vessels of the Chest Cavity

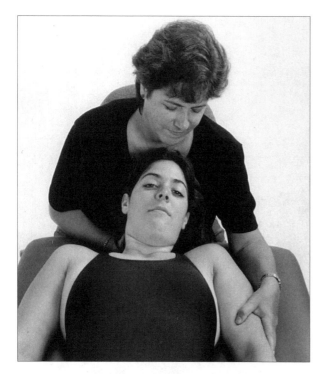

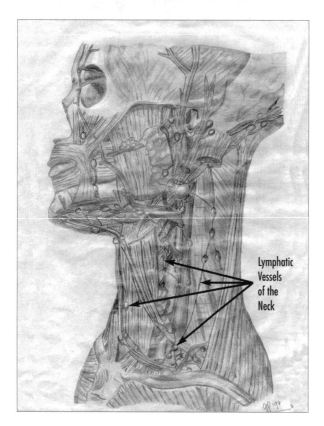

Lymphatic
Vessels
of the
Neck

Lymph/5: Neck Lymphatic Vessels
(Netter's plate #66)
(Bilateral)

TENDER POINT

C5, on the transverse process, at the superior aspect, 1 cm medial from lateral edge.

TREATMENT

- Supine.
- Flexion of neck 20 degrees.
- Rotation of neck to the ipsilateral side 25 degrees.
- Side bending of neck to the ipsilateral side 15 degrees.
- Shoulder girdle elevation (shoulder shrugging) 20 degrees.
  (no protraction of shoulder girdles)

GOAL

Release of the smooth muscles of the lymphatic vessels of the neck.

INTEGRATIVE MANUAL THERAPY™

The value of this technique cannot be over-emphasized. Because approximately one third (1/3) of all lymph nodes are in the neck region, especially the lateral neck, the benefit of reduction of hypertonicity of lymph vessel muscles in this region is enormous. This technique can be used on all clients with any form of edema, neck pain and dysfunction, myofascial disorders, and speech and swallowing problems. This technique would be beneficial for someone with a cold or flu, because of the enhanced immune effects. All systemic diseases can benefit from this technique, which can be repeated daily or weekly for the immune benefits.

Lymph/6: Facial Lymphatic Vessels

(Netter's plate #66, 67)
(Bilateral)

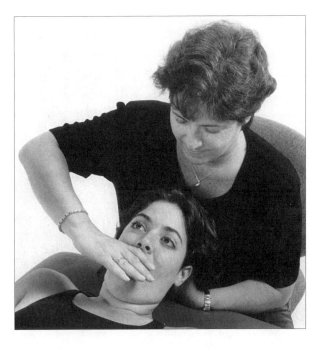

TENDER POINT

On the superior surface of zygoma, 1 inch medial to the temporo-zygomatic suture.

TREATMENT

- Supine.
- Neck flexion to 20 degrees.
- Chin tuck with over pressure on maxilla.
- Stabilize the cranial vault by holding occiput.
- Laterally glide the facial bones to the ipsilateral side with pressure from hand/hold on maxilla with 5 grams of force.

GOAL

Release of the smooth muscles of the facial lymphatic vessels.

INTEGRATIVE MANUAL THERAPY™

This technique is good for treatment of mild swelling of the face, after trauma and burns, and after surgery. There are no contraindications or precautions with this technique.

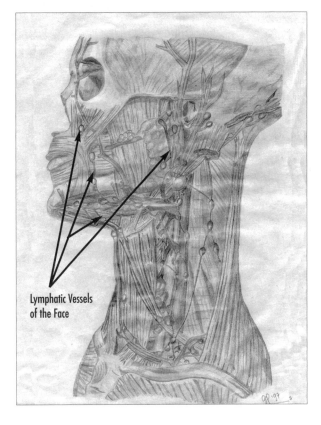

Lymphatic Vessels of the Face

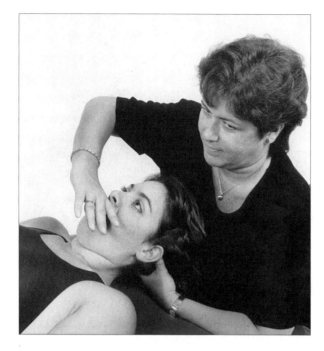

Lymph/7: Cranium and IntraCranial Lymphatic Vessels

TENDER POINT

In the suboccipital space, 1 inch lateral from midline, 1 cm anterior from outer parameter, on inferior aspect of occipital bone on the ipsilateral side.

TREATMENT

- Supine.
- Flex neck 20 degrees.
- Chin tuck with over pressure (press on maxilla, not mandible, to attain over pressure).
- Transverse glide of occiput to the ipsilateral side of the Tender Point with over pressure of 1 lb. force.

GOAL

Release of the smooth muscles of the lymphatic vessels of the cranium and IntraCranium.

INTEGRATIVE MANUAL THERAPY™

This technique integrates well with cranial therapy. Severe, mild, chronic, and acute head injuries respond well to this technique. *The results are best when Advanced Strain and Counterstrain is first performed to the diaphragms, especially the Thoracic Inlet and Cranial Diaphragm techniques.* Stroke patients may respond well with this approach also, especially when treated during the early acute phase.

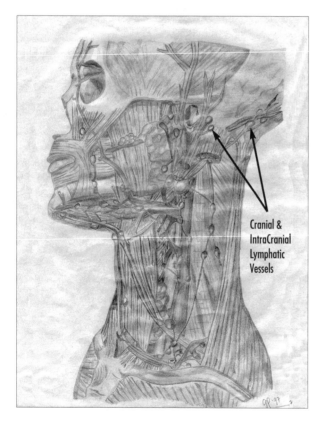

Cranial & IntraCranial Lymphatic Vessels

CHAPTER 12

ADVANCED STRAIN AND COUNTERSTRAIN FOR ARTERIES
Lower Extremities

Art/LE1: Iliac Arteries
(Netter's plate #247)
(Bilateral)

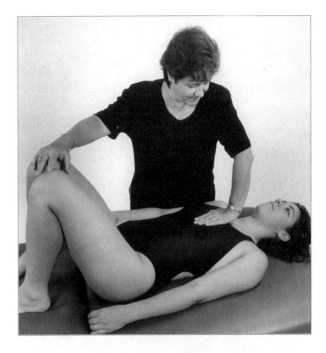

TENDER POINT

Inferior pubic symphysis.

TREATMENT

- Supine.
- Hips and knees bent.
- Knees are touching.
- Feet and heels are separated, acetabular distance apart, touching buttock.
- Tibia are internally rotated.
- Over-pressure on the sternal angle (sternal angle is between manubrium and body of sternum) in a posterior direction.
- Over-pressure on the sternal angle (sternal angle is between manubrium and body of sternum) in an inferior direction.

GOAL

Release of the smooth muscles of the iliac arteries.

INTEGRATIVE MANUAL THERAPY™

This technique is excellent for wound healing of the feet in diabetics. There are good results with peripheral neuropathy to decrease the pain of claudications. All fascial dysfunction, scar tissue, burns will improve with this technique, which may be performed for several repetitions.

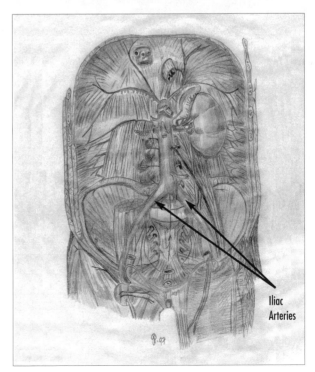

Iliac Arteries

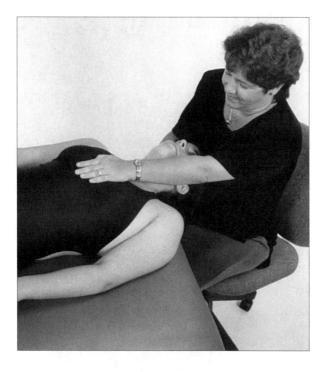

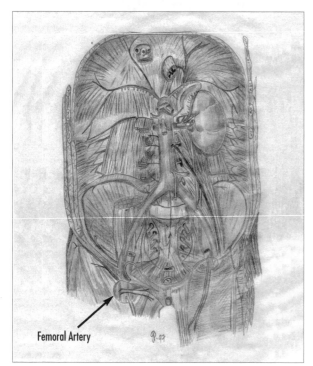

Femoral Artery

Art/LE2: Proximal Femoral Arteries
(Netter's plate #247)
(Bilateral)

TENDER POINT

Inferior pubic Symphysis (This Tender Point also reflects muscle spasm of the Iliac artery.)

TREATMENT

- Supine.
- Trunk side bending to the ipsilateral side 20 degrees,
- Cervical extension 20 degrees (head off bed).
- Both hips and knees flexed.
- Knees are touching.
- Feet and heels are separated on bed, acetabular distance apart.
- Heels are touching buttock.
- Tibia internally rotated.
- Over-pressure on the sternal angle (sternal angle is between manubrium and body of sternum) in a posterior direction.
- Over-pressure on the sternal angle (sternal angle is between manubrium and body of sternum) in an inferior direction.

GOAL

Release of the smooth muscles of the proximal femoral artery.

INTEGRATIVE MANUAL THERAPY™

This technique is excellent for wound healing of the feet in diabetics. There are good results with peripheral neuropathy and to decrease pain of claudications. All fascial dysfunction, scar tissue, burns will improve with this technique, which may be performed for several repetitions.

CHAPTER 13

ADVANCED STRAIN AND COUNTERSTRAIN FOR ARTERIES
Upper Extremities

Art/UE1: Arteries of the Arm
(Netter's plate #408, 446)
(Bilateral)

TENDER POINT

At the upper arm, 2 inches superior to the medial aspect of the medial epicondyle.

TREATMENT

- Sitting.
- Shoulder flexion to 90 degrees.
- Shoulder abduction to 90 degrees.
- Elbow flexion to 50 degrees.
- Forearm supination to 5 degrees.
- Wrist extension to 15 degrees.
- Fingers extended (neutral).

GOAL

Release of the smooth muscles of the arteries of the arm.

INTEGRATIVE MANUAL THERAPY™

This technique is good for the patient with arterial blood flow problems, observed as: decreased radial pulse, blue and mottled color of the skin, scarring (which would not occur if there was excellent arterial flow).Often there is excessive perspiration which indicates compromised arterial flow.

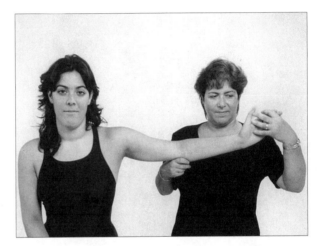

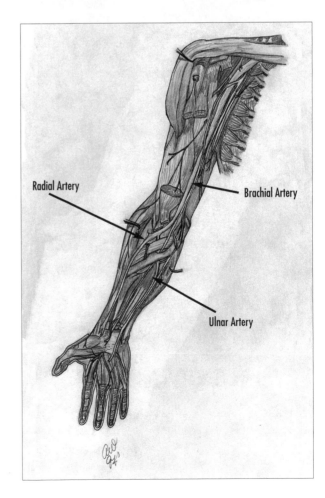

Radial Artery

Brachial Artery

Ulnar Artery

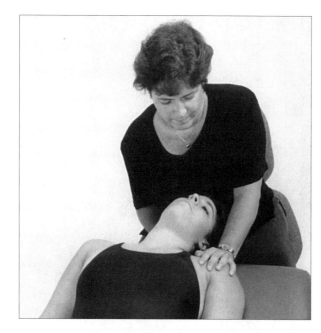

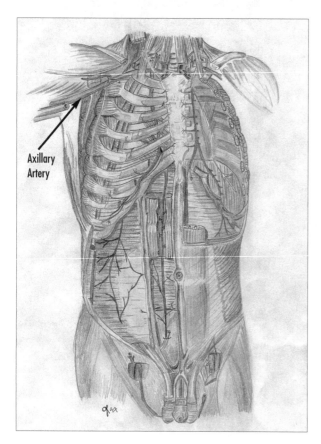

Axillary
Artery

Art/UE2: Axillary Artery
(Netter's plate #402, 404, 446)
(Bilateral)

TENDER POINT

1 inch lateral to Bregma (Axillary artery Tender Point on cranium).

TREATMENT

- Supine.
- Neck extension to 20 degrees.
- Neck rotation to 30 degrees to the ipsilateral side.
- Neck side bending to 25 degrees to the ipsilateral side.
- Shoulder girdle depression, with 1 lb. of force.
- Shoulder joint at 0 degrees anatomic neutral.
- Elbow is straight.
- The forearm is neutral: 0 degrees of supination/pronation.
- Wrist extension to 30 degrees.
- Fingers are in a neutral position: extended.

GOAL

Release of the smooth muscles of the axillary artery.

INTEGRATIVE MANUAL THERAPY™

This technique will affect edema and pain in the axilla. Good results will occur after mastectomy, radiation, infection and inflammation affecting the axillary lymph nodes. Often there is compression of the axillary artery in the armpit by the humeral head when the humeral head is subluxed inferior because of hypertonicity of the latissimus dorsi. (The latissimus dorsi is the depressor muscle of the humeral head.) Jones' Strain and Counterstrain technique for the Latissimus dorsi can precede this technique.

Art/UE3: Brachial Artery

(Netter's plate #404, 408, 446)
(Bilateral)

TENDER POINT

Lateral arm, 5 inches superior to lateral epicondyle and 3/4 inch posterior.

TREATMENT

- Supine.
- Shoulder is off the edge of the bed.
- Shoulder extension to 10 degrees.
- Shoulder abduction to 30 degrees.
- Elbow is straight.
- Wrist and fingers are in a neutral position.

GOAL

Release of the smooth muscles of the brachial artery.

INTEGRATIVE MANUAL THERAPY™

There are good results observed such as: improved healing of wounds, scars and burns of the upper arm. Excellent results with all fibromyalgia-like syndromes of the upper arm, from whatever etiology.

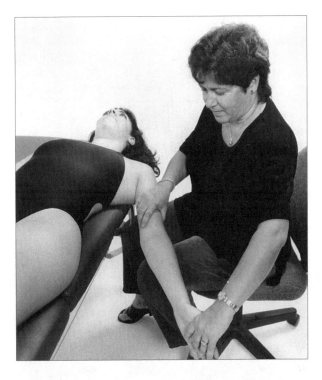

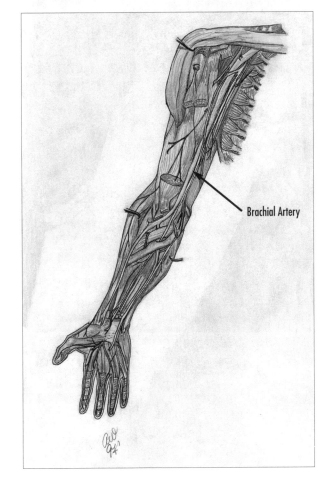

Brachial Artery

CHAPTER 14

ADVANCED STRAIN AND COUNTERSTRAIN FOR ARTERIES
Cranial and Cervical Region

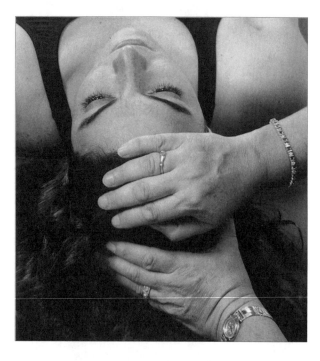

Art/Cranial1: Arteries of the Brain
(Netter's plate #130–136)
(Bilateral)

TENDER POINT

Immediately posterior to the coronal suture, 1 inch lateral from Bregma.

TREATMENT

- Supine.
- Place a hand on either side of the coronal suture.
- Coronal suture "separation": Frontal border of suture moves anterior and parietal border of suture moves posterior.
- Then side glide both sides (anterior and posterior) of the coronal suture towards the ipsilateral side of the Tender Point.

GOAL

Release of the smooth muscles of the arteries of the brain.

INTEGRATIVE MANUAL THERAPY™

This is a General Advanced Strain and Counterstrain technique, and can be performed without other techniques. (This is different from the Carotid techniques which are best performed together as a group.) This technique is best performed bilateral, to ensure fewer treatment reactions. There are good results for migraine clients who are experiencing symptoms, including auras, due to compromised arterial flow to the brain. Neck pain patients often have compromised Carotid flow secondary to musculoskeletal tensions. Use this technique for all cranial and brain dysfunction, including stroke/CVA, traumatic brain injury, anoxia to the brain, diabetes, amnesia, cerebral palsy, etc. If there are only mild signs and symptoms, this technique may eliminate most of the symptomatology secondary to compromised arterial flow to the brain.

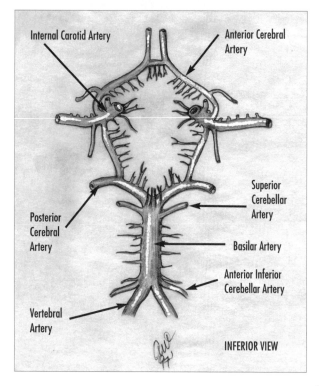

Internal Carotid Artery
Anterior Cerebral Artery
Superior Cerebellar Artery
Posterior Cerebral Artery
Basilar Artery
Anterior Inferior Cerebellar Artery
Vertebral Artery
INFERIOR VIEW

Art/Cranial2: Arteries of The Circle of Willis

(Netter's plate #133)
(Bilateral)

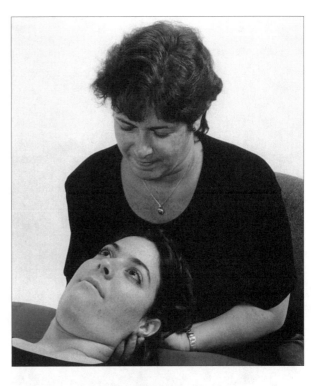

TENDER POINT

At inion, at the lateral border of inion.

TREATMENT

- Supine.
- Neck flexion to 10 degrees.
- Neck rotation to 10 degrees to the ipsilateral side.
- Neck side bending 5 degrees to the ipsilateral side.
- Compress (squeeze) occiput from occipital condyles gently with 5 grams of force.

GOAL

Release of the smooth muscles of the artery of circle of Willis.

INTEGRATIVE MANUAL THERAPY™

This Advanced Strain and Counterstrain technique is performed with the technique for the basilar artery, which is also performed bilateral, prior to treatment with the cerebral arteries techniques. PLEASE PERFORM THE CIRCLE OF WILLIS TECHNIQUE AFTER YOU HAVE PERFORMED ALL OF THE TECHNIQUES FOR ALL OF THE DIAPHRAGMS (PELVIC DIAPHRAGM, RESPIRATORY ABDOMINAL DIAPHRAGM, THORACIC INLET, AND CRANIAL DIAPHRAGM) BILATERAL. This Circle of Willis technique is specific for: all cranial and brain and spinal cord dysfunction. Brain stem disorders are occasionally dramatically improved with this technique. All craniofacial, craniomandibular, and craniocervical clients will have at least some improvement with this technique.

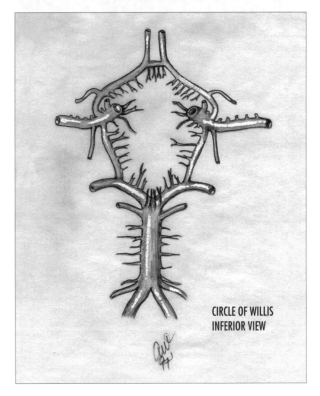

CIRCLE OF WILLIS
INFERIOR VIEW

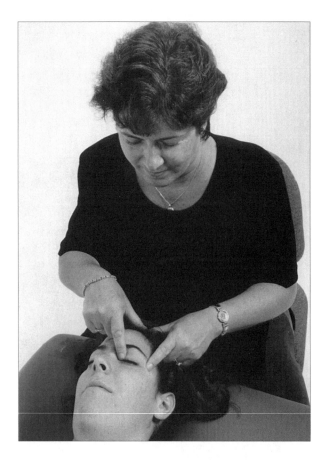

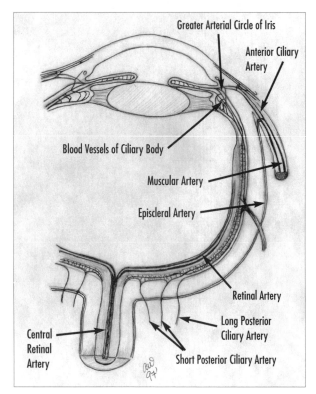

Art/Cranial3: Arteries of the Eyes

(Netter's plate #86)
(Bilateral)

TENDER POINT

At the lateral rim, just lateral to the orbit, on the posterior rim of the orbit.

TREATMENT

- Supine.
- Pressure of the lateral orbit rim, posterior to anterior/medial, with 5 grams force.
- Then push (GENTLY!! less than 1 gram of force) the eyeball towards the tender point, from a medial to a lateral direction.

GOAL

Release of the smooth muscles of the artery of eyes.

INTEGRATIVE MANUAL THERAPY™

PLEASE PERFORM THE ARTERY OF THE EYES TECHNIQUE AFTER YOU HAVE PERFORMED ALL OF THE TECHNIQUES FOR ALL OF THE DIAPHRAGMS (PELVIC DIAPHRAGM, RESPIRATORY ABDOMINAL DIAPHRAGM, THORACIC INLET, AND CRANIAL DIAPHRAGM) BILATERAL. This technique will contribute to healing of eye disease and dysfunction. Often vascular pressures secondary to arterial spasm of the eye artery contributes to: eye pain; burning of the eyes; blurred vision; diploplia; and other symptomatology. This technique can be used for all disorders, including: glaucoma, diabetes, and other diseases.

Art/Cranial4: Artery of the Hypothalamus

(Netter's plate #133)

(Bilateral)

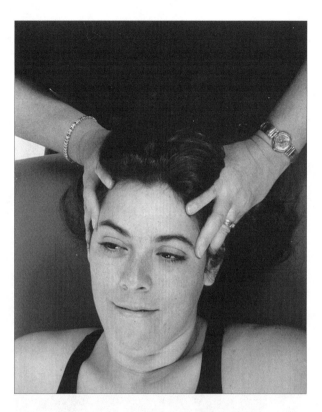

TENDER POINT

Larger tender point, over the temple, encompassing the superior and anterior suture of the sphenotemporal and sphenofrontal suture.

TREATMENT

- Supine.
- Compress medial (squeeze) both wings of the sphenoid gently with 5 grams of force.
- Maintain this compression force.
- Compress inferior both wings of the sphenoid gently with 5 grams of force.
- Neck flexion to 20 degrees.
- Neck rotation to the ipsilateral side to 30 degrees.
- Neck side bending to the ipsilateral side to 30 degrees.

GOAL

Release of the smooth muscles of the artery of the hypothalamus.

INTEGRATIVE MANUAL THERAPY™

PLEASE PERFORM THE ARTERIES OF THE HYPOTHALAMUS TECHNIQUE AFTER YOU HAVE PERFORMED ALL OF THE TECHNIQUES FOR ALL OF THE DIAPHRAGMS (PELVIC DIAPHRAGM, RESPIRATORY ABDOMINAL DIAPHRAGM, THORACIC INLET, AND CRANIAL DIAPHRAGM) BILATERAL. This technique is used for all central nervous system (brain and spinal cord) disorders which are presenting with: temperature and water balance and regulation problems; sympathetic and parasympathetic imbalance problems, including all skin color, texture, heat/cold, perspiration, and more; any brain dysfunction indicating disabilities of sinus and drainage; and more.

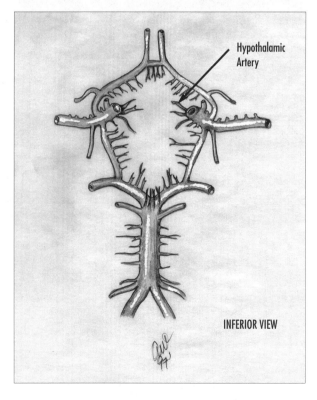

Hypothalamic Artery

INFERIOR VIEW

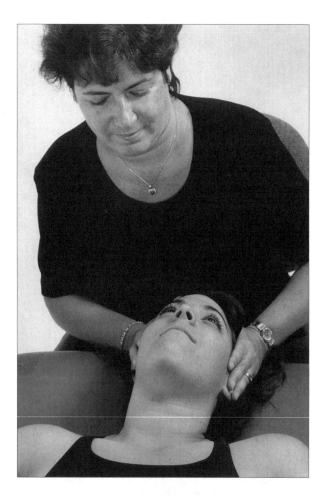

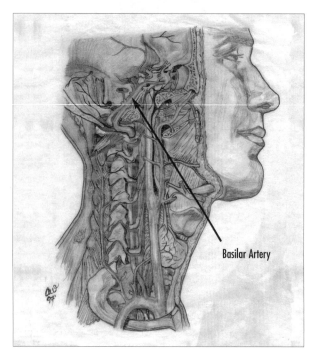

Basilar Artery

Art/Cranial5: Basilar Artery
(Netter's plate #130–136)
(Bilateral)

TENDER POINT

Posterior to occipitomastoid suture, 1 inch superior from tip of mastoid process.

TREATMENT

- Supine.
- Place both hands over patient's ears. (Cover the Temporal regions rather than the face).
- "Squeeze" gently with 5 grams force with both hands.
- Occiput extension to 5 degrees.
- Occipital side glide to the ipsilateral side.

GOAL

Release of the smooth muscles of the basilar artery.

INTEGRATIVE MANUAL THERAPY™

PLEASE PERFORM THE BASILAR ARTERY TECHNIQUE AFTER YOU HAVE PERFORMED ALL OF THE TECHNIQUES FOR ALL OF THE DIAPHRAGMS (PELVIC DIAPHRAGM, RESPIRATORY ABDOMINAL DIAPHRAGM, THORACIC INLET, AND CRANIAL DIAPHRAGM) BILATERAL. This technique is valuable, and should be performed bilateral, together with the Circle of Willis technique. This basilar artery technique together with the circle of Willis technique should be performed prior to the cerebral artery techniques. This Advanced Strain and Counterstrain technique is specific for: brain stem disorders; cerebellar dysfunction; cranial nerve dysfunction. These may manifest as: balance and equilibrium dysfunction; speech and swallowing problems; respiratory dysfunction; visual problems; hearing loss and tinnitus; torticollis; hypertonicity; sleep disorders including sleep apnea; and more. This technique is extremely valuable for clients experiencing Transient Ischemic Attacks.

Art/Cranial6: Carotid–Common Carotid Artery

(Netter's plate #29, 63,70, 130, 131)
(Bilateral)

TENDER POINT

Lateral aspect of C5 transverse process, anterior 2/3 inch.

TREATMENT

- Supine.
- Neck flexion to 30 degrees.
- Neck rotation to 20 degrees to ipsilateral side.
- No neck side bending.
- Compression through the head. Hand is on the parietal, ipsilateral side. Inferior compression through C5 transverse process with 5 grams force.
- Push C4 in a lateral glide towards the contralateral side.

GOAL

Release of the smooth muscles of the common carotid artery.

INTEGRATIVE MANUAL THERAPY™

PLEASE PERFORM THE COMMON CAROTID ARTERY TECHNIQUE AFTER YOU HAVE PERFORMED ALL OF THE TECHNIQUES FOR ALL OF THE DIAPHRAGMS (PELVIC DIAPHRAGM, RESPIRATORY ABDOMINAL DIAPHRAGM, THORACIC INLET, AND CRANIAL DIAPHRAGM) BILATERAL. Advanced Strain and Counterstrain is best performed bilateral, and often there are less treatment reactions when all of the carotid techniques are performed, rather than just a few. There are often exceptional results for migraine clients who are experiencing symptoms , including auras, due to compromised arterial flow to the brain. Neck pain patients often have compromised Carotid flow secondary to musculoskeletal tensions. Use this technique for all cranial and brain dysfunction, including: stroke/CVA, traumatic brain injury, anoxia to the brain, diabetes, amnesia, cerebral palsy, etc.

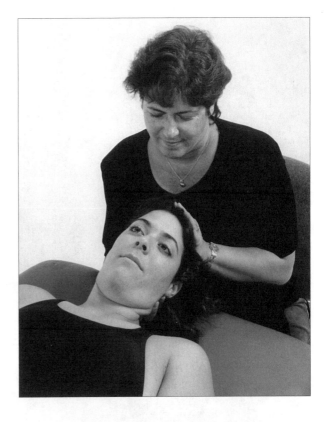

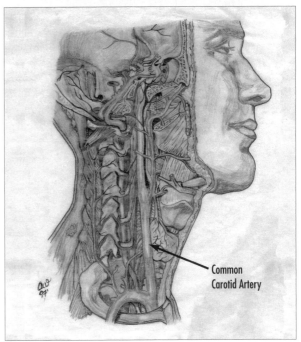

Common Carotid Artery

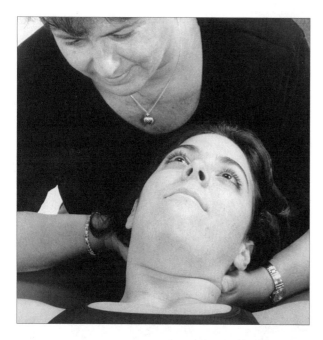

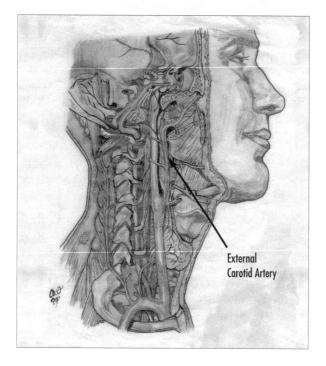

External
Carotid Artery

Art/Cranial7: Carotid–External Carotid Artery

(Netter's plate #29, 63, 70, 130, 131, 216)
(Bilateral)

TENDER POINT

Lateral aspect of C3 transverse process, 1 inch anterior.

TREATMENT

- Supine.
- Neck flexion to 20 degrees.
- Neck rotation to 10 degrees to the ipsilateral side.
- Neck side bending to 20 degrees to the ipsilateral side.
- Push C3 to a lateral glide towards the ipsilateral side with 5 grams of force.

GOAL

Release of the smooth muscles of the external carotid artery.

INTEGRATIVE MANUAL THERAPY™

PLEASE PERFORM THE EXTERNAL CAROTID ARTERY TECHNIQUE AFTER YOU HAVE PERFORMED ALL OF THE TECHNIQUES FOR ALL OF THE DIAPHRAGMS (PELVIC DIAPHRAGM, RESPIRATORY ABDOMINAL DIAPHRAGM, THORACIC INLET, AND CRANIAL DIAPHRAGM) BILATERAL. Advanced Strain and Counterstrain is best performed bilateral, and often there are less treatment reactions when all of the Carotid techniques are performed, rather than just a few. There are often exceptional results for migraine clients who are experiencing symptoms , including auras, due to compromised arterial flow to the brain. Neck pain patients often have compromised carotid flow secondary to musculoskeletal tensions. Use this technique for all cranial and brain dysfunction, including: stroke/CVA, traumatic brain injury, anoxia to the brain, diabetes, amnesia, cerebral palsy, etc.

Art/Cranial8: Carotid—Internal Carotid Artery

(Netter's plate #29, 63, 70, 130, 131, 216)
(Bilateral)

TENDER POINT

On lung, through thoracic inlet: Finger access via sternal notch on most superior and medial aspect of lung.

TREATMENT

- Supine.
- Neck flexion to 50 degrees.
- Neck rotation to 30 degrees to the ipsilateral side.
- Neck side bending to 20 degrees to the ipsilateral side
- Compress inferior from sternal notch (use thenar eminence) with 5 grams of force.

GOAL

Release of the smooth muscles of the internal carotid artery.

INTEGRATIVE MANUAL THERAPY™

Advanced Strain and Counterstrain is best performed bilateral, and often there are less treatment reactions when all of the Carotid techniques are performed, rather than just a few. There are exceptional results for real migraine clients who are experiencing symptoms, including auras, due to compromised arterial flow to the brain. Neck pain patients often have compromised carotid flow secondary to musculoskeletal tensions. Use this technique for all cranial and brain dysfunction, including: stroke/CVA, traumatic brain injury, anoxia to the brain, diabetes, amnesia, cerebral palsy, etc.

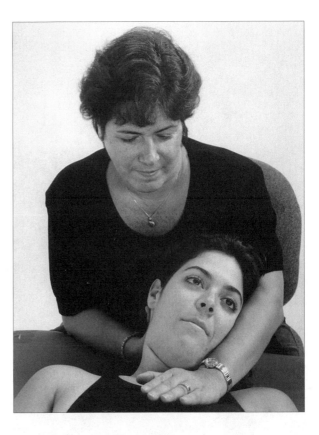

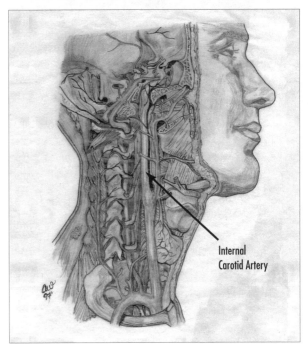

Internal Carotid Artery

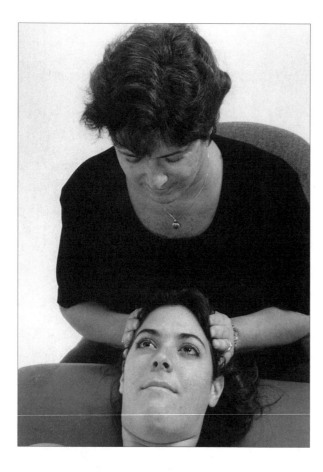

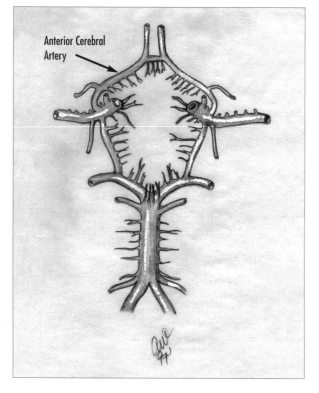

Anterior Cerebral Artery

Art/Cranial9: Cerebral— Anterior Cerebral Artery

(Netter's plate #131–135)
(Bilateral)

TENDER POINT

On temporal, 1 inch anterior from the occipito-mastoid suture and 2 inches superior from tip of mastoid process.

TREATMENT

- Supine.
- Compress (squeeze) superior aspects of temporal bone gently with 5 grams of force.
- Then neck flexion to 30 degrees.
- (Both right and left sides are treated in this position.)

GOAL

Release of the smooth muscles of the anterior cerebral artery.

INTEGRATIVE MANUAL THERAPY™

The cerebral arteries techniques are wonderful tools for manual practitioners. There are exceptional results with these techniques. PLEASE PERFORM ALL OF THE CEREBRAL ARTERY TECHNIQUES BILATERAL. PLEASE PERFORM ALL OF THE CEREBRAL ARTERY TECHNIQUES AFTER YOU HAVE PERFORMED THE TECHNIQUES FOR THE BASILAR ARTERY AND THE CIRCLE OF WILLIS BILATERAL. PLEASE PERFORM ALL OF THE CEREBRAL ARTERY TECHNIQUES AFTER YOU HAVE PERFORMED ALL OF THE TECHNIQUES FOR ALL OF THE DIAPHRAGMS (PELVIC DIAPHRAGM, RESPIRATORY ABDOMINAL DIAPHRAGM, THORACIC INLET, AND CRANIAL DIAPHRAGM) BILATERAL. These cerebral artery techniques may attain remarkable results for all central nervous system (brain and spinal cord) patients, including: traumatic brain injury and closed head injury, cerebral palsy, anoxic brain damage, stroke/CVA, toxic brain and spinal cord damage from radiation and metal toxicity and more, and all other CNS disturbances. This Advanced Strain and Counterstrain technique for the anterior cerebral artery will be specific for: cognitive problems, visual impairments, learning disabilities, mental retardation, judgement disorders, dislexias, and other frontal lobe disturbances.

Art/Cranial10: Cerebral— Middle Cerebral Artery

(Netter's plate #131–135)
(Bilateral)

TENDER POINT

On temporal, 2 inches anterior from occipito-mastoid suture, one and one-half (1½) inches superior from tip of mastoid process.

TREATMENT

- Supine.
- Compress (squeeze) lateral aspects of coronal sutures gently with 5 grams of force.
- Neck flexion to 20 degrees.
- Neck rotation to 15 degrees to the ipsilateral side.

GOAL

Release of the smooth muscles of the middle cerebral artery.

INTEGRATIVE MANUAL THERAPY™

The cerebral arteries techniques are wonderful tools for manual practitioners. There are exceptional results with these techniques. PLEASE PERFORM ALL OF THE CEREBRAL ARTERY TECHNIQUES BILATERAL. PLEASE PERFORM ALL OF THE CEREBRAL ARTERY TECHNIQUES AFTER YOU HAVE PERFORMED THE TECHNIQUES FOR THE BASILAR ARTERY AND THE CIRCLE OF WILLIS BILATERAL. PLEASE PERFORM ALL OF THE CEREBRAL ARTERY TECHNIQUES AFTER YOU HAVE PERFORMED ALL OF THE TECHNIQUES FOR ALL OF THE DIAPHRAGMS (PELVIC DIAPHRAGM, RESPIRATORY ABDOMINAL DIAPHRAGM, THORACIC INLET, AND CRANIAL DIAPHRAGM) BILATERAL. These cerebral artery techniques may attain remarkable results for all central nervous system (brain and spinal cord) patients, including: traumatic brain injury and closed head injury, cerebral palsy, anoxic brain damage, stroke/CVA, toxic brain and spinal cord damage from radiation and metal toxicity and more, and all other CNS disturbances. This Advanced Strain and Counterstrain technique for the middle cerebral artery is specific for: stroke/CVA clients, TIA (transient is-

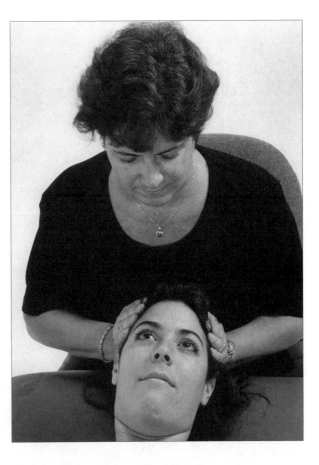

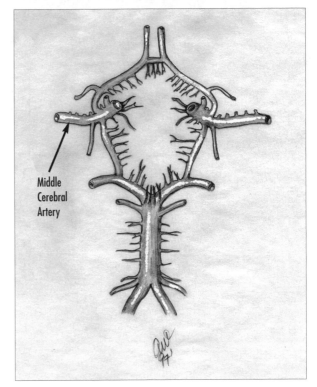

Middle Cerebral Artery

chemic attacks), seizures disorders (of all natures), brain injuries (traumatic and anoxic), basal ganglia and thalamus disorders, and any and all other CNS dysfunction.

Art/Cranial11: Cerebral— Posterior Cerebral Artery

(Netter's plate #131–135)
(Bilateral)

TENDER POINT

On temporal, one (1) inch anterior from the occipitomastoid suture and 2 inches superior from the meatus.

TREATMENT

- Supine.
- Compress (squeeze) posterior/superior aspects of temporoparietal sutures gently with 5 grams force.
- Then "lift head" (translation rather than flexion) towards the ceiling with 1 pound of force.
- Neck rotation 10 degrees to the ipsilateral side.

GOAL

Release of the smooth muscles of the posterior cerebral artery.

INTEGRATIVE MANUAL THERAPY™

The cerebral arteries techniques are wonderful tools for manual practitioners. There are exceptional results with these techniques. PLEASE PERFORM ALL OF THE CEREBRAL ARTERY TECHNIQUES BILATERAL. PLEASE PERFORM ALL OF THE CEREBRAL ARTERY TECHNIQUES AFTER YOU HAVE PERFORMED THE TECHNIQUES FOR THE BASILAR ARTERY AND THE CIRCLE OF WILLIS BILATERAL. PLEASE PERFORM ALL OF THE CEREBRAL ARTERY TECHNIQUES AFTER YOU HAVE PERFORMED ALL OF THE TECHNIQUES FOR ALL OF THE DIAPHRAGMS (PELVIC DIAPHRAGM, RESPIRATORY ABDOMINAL DIAPHRAGM, THORACIC INLET, AND CRANIAL DIAPHRAGM) BILATERAL. These cerebral artery techniques may attain remarkable results for all central nervous system (brain and spinal cord) patients, including: traumatic brain injury and closed head injury, cerebral palsy, anoxic brain damage, stroke/CVA, toxic brain and spinal cord damage

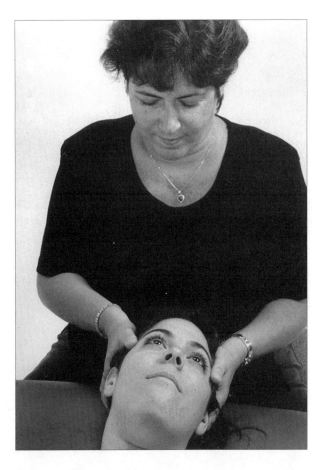

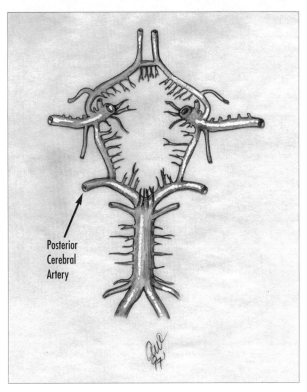

Posterior Cerebral Artery

from radiation and metal toxicity and more, and all other CNS disturbances. This Advanced Strain and Counterstrain technique for the posterior cerebral artery is specific for: visual impairments, visual perceptual and visual spatial problems, equilibrium and balance and coordination disorders, spinal cord injuries, brain stem problems of the medulla and pons, spasticity secondary to dysfunction at the pyramidal tracts decussation often seen as diplegia, all cranial nerve problems (for example vagus problems resulting in projectile vomiting; glossopharyngeal and hypoglossal problems resulting in speech and swallowing impairments; spinal accessory problems causing torticollis; oculomotor, trochlea, and abducens problems causing ocular muscle disorders; and more.)

Art/Cranial12: Middle Meningeal Artery

(Netter's plate #95)
(Bilateral)

TENDER POINT

Suboccipital space, one-and-a-half (1½) inches medial to the tip of the mastoid process. Compress superior for tender point.

TREATMENT

- Supine.
- Lateral glide of occiput to the ipsilateral side.
- Hyperextend occiput on atlas without any extension of C1 through C7.
- Neck rotation to 25 degrees to the ipsilateral side.

GOAL

Release of the smooth muscles of the middle meningeal artery.

INTEGRATIVE MANUAL THERAPY™

PLEASE PERFORM THE MIDDLE MENINGEAL ARTERY TECHNIQUE AFTER YOU HAVE PERFORMED ALL OF THE TECHNIQUES FOR ALL OF THE DIAPHRAGMS (PELVIC DIAPHRAGM, RESPIRATORY ABDOMINAL DIAPHRAGM, THORACIC INLET, AND CRANIAL DIAPHRAGM) BILATERAL. This technique can be used for all spinal patients, whether for back pain relief or spinal cord injury. Often there is low grade arachnoiditis after trauma, after surgery, after disease. This technique is excellent for treatment of arachnoiditis. Occasionally spinal cord fibrosis is perceived when there is really contraction of the spinal cord around the meningeal artery. This technique can be performed prior to cranial and craniosacral therapy, and prior to neurofascial release (Weiselfish-Giammatteo).

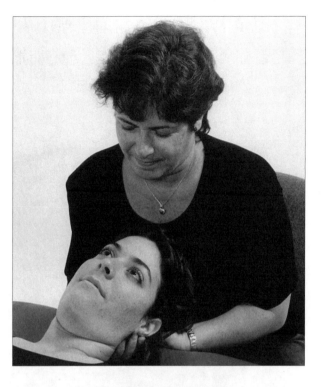

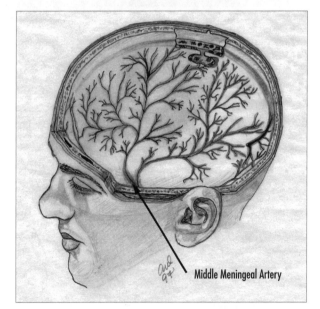

Middle Meningeal Artery

CHAPTER 15

ADVANCED STRAIN AND COUNTERSTRAIN FOR ARTERIES
Cardiopulmonary System

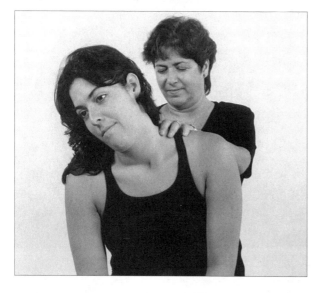

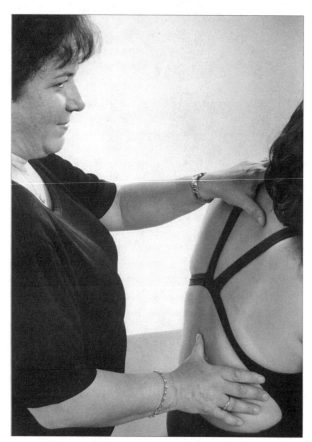

Art/Cardio1: Aorta

(Netter's plate #216–221, 247–249, 333)
(Unilateral)

TENDER POINT

Left mid clavicular line, on the 4th rib, 1 inch medial. Access the hypomobility.

TREATMENT

- Sitting.
- Trunk rotation right 10 degrees.
- Trunk side bending right 10-15 degrees.
- Cervical rotation to the right 10 degrees.
- Cervical side bending to the right 5 degrees.
- Assess mobility: Do superior mobility test of T2, T3, and T4. Choose the vertebra which is most hypomobile in superior glide.
- Over-pressure T2 or T3 or T4 spinous process into flexion (superior glide). Flex the hypomobile vertebra.
- Superior lift of the spinous process of L3.

GOAL

Release of the smooth muscles of the aorta.

INTEGRATIVE MANUAL THERAPY™

PLEASE PERFORM THE CARDIOPULMONARY TECHNIQUES AFTER YOU HAVE PERFORMED ALL OF THE TECHNIQUES FOR ALL OF THE DIAPHRAGMS (PELVIC DIAPHRAGM, RESPIRATORY ABDOMINAL DIAPHRAGM, THORACIC INLET, AND CRANIAL DIAPHRAGM) BILATERAL. This amazing technique will facilitate multiple changes in the client with somatic disorders. The body protects arteries because of the permeability of the membranes. If there is dysfunction of an artery, the hypertonicity of the musculature of that artery will affect the permeability and the fragility of the membrane. The body will provide protection. This protection is for prevention of further injury to the artery. The body will provide containment: with reflexive and protective muscle spasm and fascial tightening, and limitations of ranges of motion. For example, when the muscles of the aorta are in a state of hypertonicity, the left shoulder girdle will be in a reflexive state of protraction so that horizontal abduction and extension and external rotation is inhibited. If the aorta is in a 'critical' state, horizontal abduction, extension and external rotation of the left shoulder girdle would provoke more tension on the aorta. Hold this technique beyond the one minute of Advanced Strain and Counterstrain during the De-Facilitated Fascial Release; the results will be extraordinary. Measure pulse and blood pressure as pre-and post-testing for all cardio-pulmonary and cardio-vascular clients. Observe the immediate increase in ranges of motion after this technique, including: all left shoulder girdle and shoulder joint movements; cervical motions, especially extension and right rotation and right side bending; thoracic motions, especially extension, right rotation and right side bending. There will often be a change in total body edema, which was secondary to extracellular edema from tension surrounding the aorta. Occasionally heartburn will subside due to decreases in tension of the oesophagus/aorta junction, which appears to be associated with acid production (indeed, there is often a decrease in gout symptomotology). Observe all of the body's signs and symptoms prior to the techniques, in order to appreciate the changes. This technique is best performed after Jones Strain and Counterstrain for the second depressed rib (which eliminates the hypertonicity of the pectoralis minor), followed by the 3-Planar Fascial Fulcrum Technique (Weiselfish-Giammatteo, Myofascial Release) for the left clavipectoral region. Use this technique for all left TOS (thoracic outlet syndrome) and RSD (reflex sympathetic dystrophy), and all left arm angina pectoris symptoms. There are no contraindications for this technique.

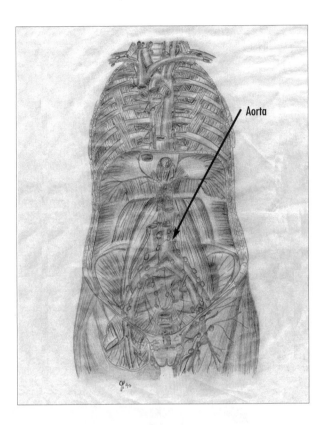

Aorta

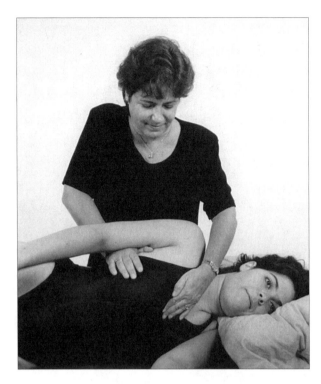

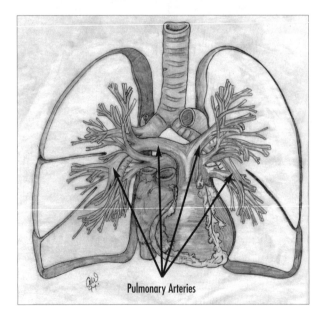

Pulmonary Arteries

Art/Cardio2: Arteries of the Lung
(Netter's plate #193–199)
(Bilateral)

TENDER POINT

Just lateral to the 4th sternochondral joint line.

TREATMENT

- Side lying on the contralateral side.
- Compress on the 4th sternochondral joint in a posterior direction.
- Compress on the 4th sternochondral joint in an inferior direction.
- Press on the lateral rib cage, in a lateral to medial direction, with 3 lbs. of pressure.

GOAL

Release of the smooth muscles of the artery of the lung.

INTEGRATIVE MANUAL THERAPY™

PLEASE PERFORM THE CARDIOPULMONARY TECHNIQUES AFTER YOU HAVE PERFORMED ALL OF THE TECHNIQUES FOR ALL OF THE DIAPHRAGMS (PELVIC DIAPHRAGM, RESPIRATORY ABDOMINAL DIAPHRAGM, THORACIC INLET, AND CRANIAL DIAPHRAGM) BILATERAL. This technique will affect all cardiovascular and respiratory ailments. There may be exceptionally good results with asthma and bronchial spasm, because it appears that the chest contracts around these arteries for protection when they are in a state of hypertonicity. Rib expansion may increase dramatically. Necrosis of the lungs because of chronic smoking, radiation, surgery resulting in vascular tissue damage, and other invasive projections into the lungs may begin to heal when this technique is repeated several times during a six to twelve month period of time. There are no contraindications with this technique. It can be used immediately status post cardiac and pulmonary surgery for improved healing.

Art/Cardio3: Intraventricular Coronary Arteries

(Netter's plate #204-215)
(Bilateral)

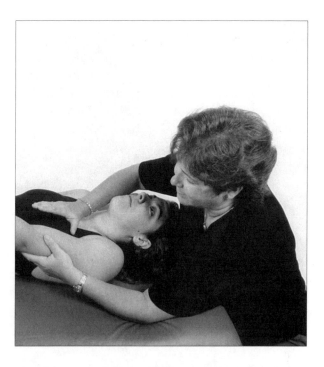

TENDER POINT

2nd Sternochondral joint, on the joint line.

TREATMENT

- Supine.
- Compress anterior to posterior on 2nd sternochondral joint line with 5 grams of force.
- Then (maintain compression) compress inferior with 5 grams of force.
- Then compress lateral towards the side of the tender point with 5 grams force.
- Maintain all above forces.
- Shoulder flexion 30 degrees with straight arm.

GOAL

Release of the smooth muscles of the intraventricular coronary arteries.

INTEGRATIVE MANUAL THERAPY™

PLEASE PERFORM THE CARDIOPULMONARY TECHNIQUES AFTER YOU HAVE PERFORMED ALL OF THE TECHNIQUES FOR ALL OF THE DIAPHRAGMS (PELVIC DIAPHRAGM, RESPIRATORY ABDOMINAL DIAPHRAGM, THORACIC INLET, AND CRANIAL DIAPHRAGM) BILATERAL. This technique should be performed bilateral. This technique will be effective for patients with pain and protective muscle spasm of the chest which is the result of compromised coronary arteries blood flow. There is no contraindication for this technique. This is a general technique for improved circulation to the heart muscle. The most easy-to-observe changes are increases in ranges of motion. After this technique there will be increased cervical, thoracic and even lumbar extension. Shoulder girdle horizontal abduction and extension will increase. There will be less protective adaptation of the body protecting the coronary arteries, so posture will improve, with less forward head and neck posture. Often there will be remarkable changes in the 'dowager's hump' presentation immediately after this technique.

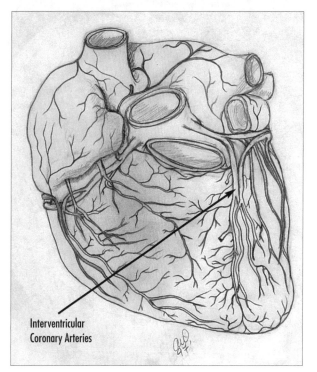

Interventricular
Coronary Arteries

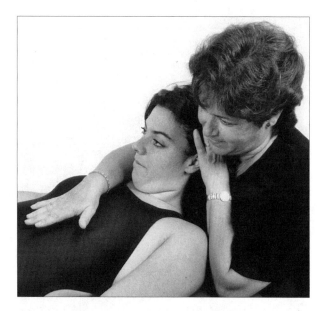

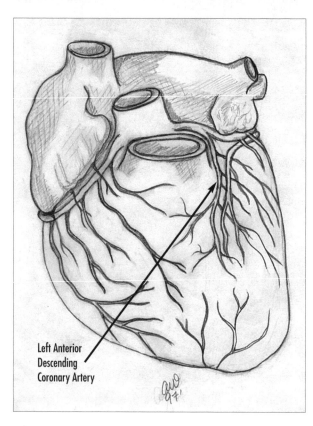

Left Anterior
Descending
Coronary Artery

Art/Cardio4: Left Anterior Descending Coronary Artery

(Netter's plate #204–215)
(Unilateral)

TENDER POINT

On left 7th intercostal space (between 7th and 8th ribs), 4 inches lateral (left) from the left sternum border.

TREATMENT

- Supine.
- Flexion of the head, neck and trunk down the kinetic chain to the left 7th intercostal space.
- Compress over the Tender Point in a posterior direction with 5 grams of force.
- Compress over the Tender Point in a medial direction with 5 grams of force.
- Compress over the Tender Point in an inferior direction with 5 grams of force.

GOAL

Release of the smooth muscles of the left anterior descending coronary artery.

INTEGRATIVE MANUAL THERAPY™

Please perform the cardiopulmonary techniques after you have performed all techniques for all diaphragms (pelvic diaphragm, respiratory abdominal diaphragm, thoracic inlet, and cranial diaphragm) bilateral. This technique should be performed bilateral. This technique will be effective for patients with pain and protective muscle spasm of the chest which is the result of compromised coronary arteries blood flow. There is no contraindication for this technique, a general technique for improved circulation to the heart muscle. The most easy-to-observe changes are increases in ranges of motion. Afterwards there will be increased cervical, thoracic and even lumbar extension. Shoulder girdle horizontal abduction and extension will increase. There will be less protective adaptation of the body protecting the coronary arteries, so posture will improve, with less forward head and neck posture. Often there will be remarkable changes in the 'dowager's hump' presentation immediately after this technique.

Art/Cardio5: Left Coronary Arteries

(Netter's plate #204–215)
(Unilateral)

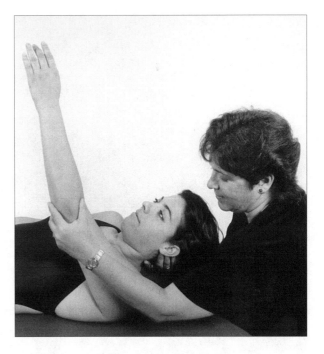

TENDER POINT

On left 3rd rib, 2 inches to the left of the sternocostal joint.

TREATMENT

- Supine.
- Left shoulder flexion to 50 degrees.
- Left horizontal adduction to 30 degrees.
- Left elbow is straight.
- Head is lifted towards ceiling (translation of head rather than flexion of neck) with a 1 lb. force.
- Compress Occipitoatlantal joints. The hand under the occiput compresses the Occiput into the Atlas.

GOAL

Release of the smooth muscles of the left coronary arteries.

INTEGRATIVE MANUAL THERAPY™

PLEASE PERFORM THE CARDIOPULMONARY TECHNIQUES AFTER YOU HAVE PERFORMED ALL OF THE TECHNIQUES FOR ALL OF THE DIAPHRAGMS (PELVIC DIAPHRAGM, RESPIRATORY ABDOMINAL DIAPHRAGM, THORACIC INLET, AND CRANIAL DIAPHRAGM) BILATERAL. This technique should be performed bilateral. This technique will be effective for patients with pain and protective muscle spasm of the chest which is the result of compromised coronary arteries blood flow. There is no contraindication for this technique; it is a general technique for improved circulation to the heart muscle. The most easy-to-observe changes are increases in ranges of motion. After this technique there will be increased cervical, thoracic and even lumbar extension. Shoulder girdle horizontal abduction and extension will increase. There will be less protective adaptation of the body protecting the coronary arteries, so posture will improve, with less forward head and neck posture. Often there will be remarkable changes in the 'dowager's hump' presentation immediately after this technique.

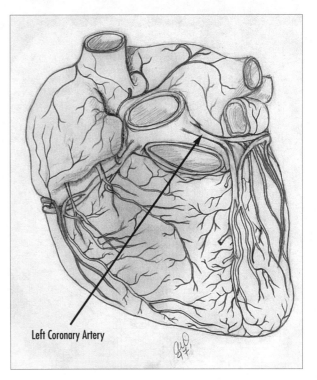

Left Coronary Artery

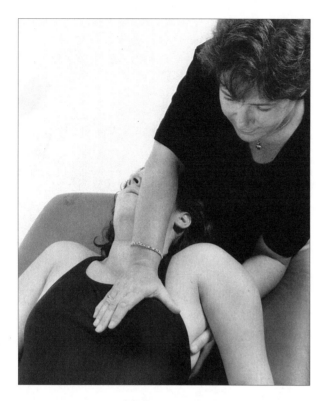

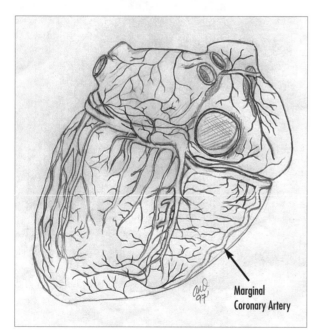

Marginal
Coronary Artery

Art/Cardio6: Marginal Coronary Arteries
(Netter's plate #204–215)
(Bilateral)

TENDER POINT

At the 3rd intercostal space, 2 inches lateral from the sternum border.

TREATMENT

- Supine.
- Place a hand on the posterior-lateral border of the upper rib cage, on the ipsilateral side.
- Lift the rib cage towards the ceiling (anterior), 1 inch off the table.
- Then compress on the ipsilateral Tender Point in a posterior direction with 5 grams of force.
- Compress on the ipsilateral Tender Point in a medial direction with 5 grams of force.

GOAL

Release of the smooth muscles of the marginal coronary artery.

INTEGRATIVE MANUAL THERAPY™

PLEASE PERFORM THE CARDIOPULMONARY TECHNIQUES AFTER YOU HAVE PERFORMED ALL OF THE TECHNIQUES FOR ALL OF THE DIAPHRAGMS (PELVIC DIAPHRAGM, RESPIRATORY ABDOMINAL DIAPHRAGM, THORACIC INLET, AND CRANIAL DIAPHRAGM) BILATERAL. This technique should be performed bilateral. This technique will be effective for patients with pain and protective muscle spasm of the chest which is the result of compromised coronary arteries blood flow. There is no contraindication for this technique, and is a general technique for improved circulation to the heart muscle. The most easy-to-observe changes are increases in ranges of motion. After this technique there will be increased cervical, thoracic and even lumbar extension. Shoulder girdle horizontal abduction and extension will increase. There will be less protective adaptation of the body protecting the coronary arteries, so posture will improve, with less forward head and neck posture. Often there will be remarkable changes in the 'dowager's hump' presentation immediately after this technique.

Art/Cardio7: Posterior Descending Coronary Arteries

(Netter's plate #204–216)
(Bilateral)

TENDER POINT

At the 6th rib, 3 inches lateral from the sternum border.

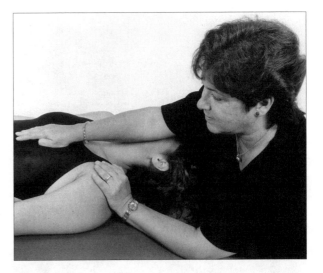

TREATMENT

- Supine.
- Compress the ipsilateral shoulder girdle inferior with a hand on the superior aspect (over the acromion).
- Compress the ipsilateral shoulder girdle medial with 5 grams of force.
- Then compress over the ipsilateral Tender Point in a posterior direction with 5 grams of force.

GOAL

Release of the smooth muscles of the posterior descending coronary arteries.

INTEGRATIVE MANUAL THERAPY™

PLEASE PERFORM THE CARDIOPULMONARY TECHNIQUES AFTER YOU HAVE PERFORMED ALL OF THE TECHNIQUES FOR ALL OF THE DIAPHRAGMS (PELVIC DIAPHRAGM, RESPIRATORY ABDOMINAL DIAPHRAGM, THORACIC INLET, AND CRANIAL DIAPHRAGM) BILATERAL. This technique should be performed bilateral. This technique will be effective for patients with pain and protective muscle spasm of the chest which is the result of compromised coronary arteries blood flow. There is no contraindication for this technique, and is a general technique for improved circulation to the heart muscle. The most easy-to-observe changes are increases in ranges of motion. After this technique there will be increased cervical, thoracic and even lumbar extension. Shoulder girdle horizontal abduction and extension will increase. There will be less protective adaptation of the body protecting the coronary arteries, so posture will improve, with less forward head and neck posture. Often there will be remarkable changes in the 'dowager's hump' presentation immediately after this technique.

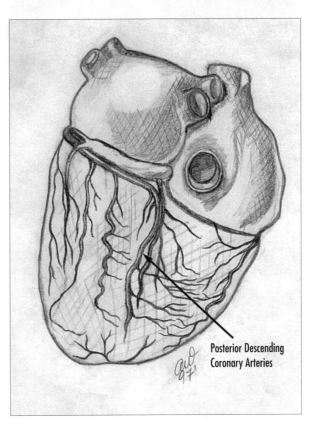

Posterior Descending Coronary Arteries

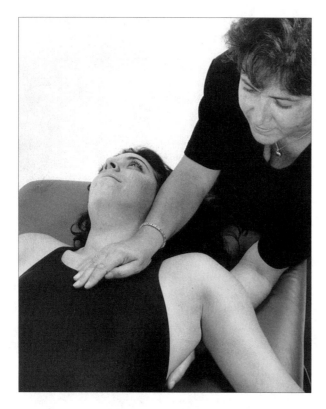

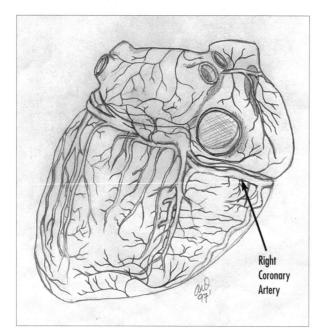

Right
Coronary
Artery

Art/Cardio8: Right Coronary Artery

(Netter's plate #204–215)
(Unilateral)

TENDER POINT

Right subclavius, middle of muscle, underneath (posterior to) the right clavicle.

TREATMENT

- Supine.
- Compress on the right subclavius muscle (over the Tender Point) in a posterior direction with 5 grams of force.
- Then lift the heart from behind (posterior to anterior), with a hand underneath the body, about 1 inch off the table.

GOAL

Release of the smooth muscles of the right coronary artery.

INTEGRATIVE MANUAL THERAPY™

PLEASE PERFORM THE CARDIOPULMONARY TECHNIQUES AFTER YOU HAVE PERFORMED ALL OF THE TECHNIQUES FOR ALL OF THE DIAPHRAGMS (PELVIC DIAPHRAGM, RESPIRATORY ABDOMINAL DIAPHRAGM, THORACIC INLET, AND CRANIAL DIAPHRAGM) BILATERAL. This technique should be performed bilateral. This technique will be effective for patients with pain and protective muscle spasm of the chest which is the result of compromised coronary arteries blood flow. There is no contraindication for this technique, and is a general technique for improved circulation to the heart muscle. The most easy-to-observe changes are increases in ranges of motion. After this technique there will be increased cervical, thoracic and even lumbar extension. Shoulder girdle horizontal abduction and extension will increase. There will be less protective adaptation of the body protecting the coronary arteries, so posture will improve, with less forward head and neck posture. Often there will be remarkable changes in the 'dowager's hump' presentation immediately after this technique.

Art/Cardio9: Right Marginal Coronary Artery

(Netter's plate #204–215)
(Unilateral)

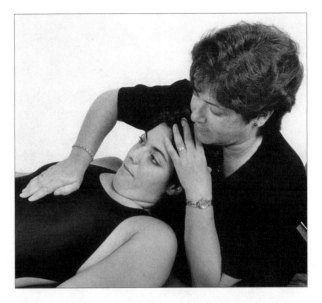

TENDER POINT

Right lung, at the medial aspect, between the 3rd and 4th sternochondral joint.

TREATMENT

- Supine.
- Neck flexion to 70 degrees.
- Neck rotation to the left 20 degrees.
- Compress over the Tender Point anterior to posterior (in a posterior direction) towards the left side with 5 grams of force.

GOAL

Release of the smooth muscles of the right marginal coronary artery.

INTEGRATIVE MANUAL THERAPY™

PLEASE PERFORM THE CARDIOPULMONARY TECHNIQUES AFTER YOU HAVE PERFORMED ALL OF THE TECHNIQUES FOR ALL OF THE DIAPHRAGMS (PELVIC DIAPHRAGM, RESPIRATORY ABDOMINAL DIAPHRAGM, THORACIC INLET, AND CRANIAL DIAPHRAGM) BILATERAL. This technique should be performed bilateral. This technique will be effective for patients with pain and protective muscle spasm of the chest which is the result of compromised coronary arteries blood flow. There is no contraindication for this technique, and is a general technique for improved circulation to the heart muscle. The most easy-to-observe changes are increases in ranges of motion. After this technique there will be increased cervical, thoracic and even lumbar extension. Shoulder girdle horizontal abduction and extension will increase. There will be less protective adaptation of the body protecting the coronary arteries, so posture will improve, with less forward head and neck posture. Often there will be remarkable changes in the 'dowager's hump' presentation immediately after this technique.

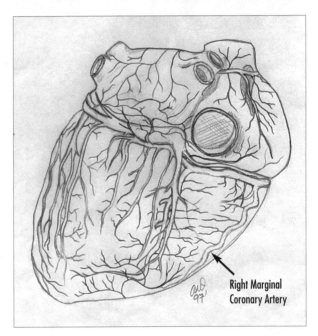

Right Marginal Coronary Artery

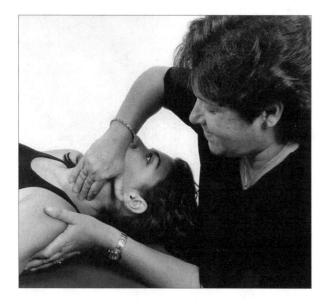

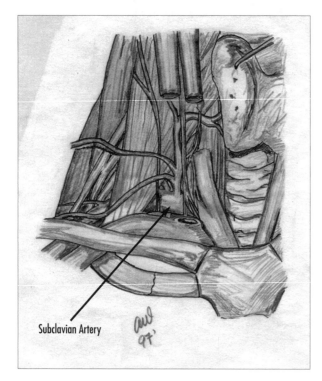

Subclavian Artery

Art/Cardio10: Subclavian Artery

(Netter's plate #26–29)
(Bilateral)

TENDER POINT

On lung, inferior to the clavicle 3 inches lateral from the middle of the sternal notch.

TREATMENT

- Supine.
- Compress and glide the humeral head in an anterior direction (posterior to anterior).
- Place the second hand anterior to the transverse process of C7.
- Press the transverse process of C7 in posterior, inferior and medial direction with 5 grams of force.

GOAL

Release of the smooth muscles of the subclavian artery. Improve respiratory function.

INTEGRATIVE MANUAL THERAPY™

Please perform the subclavian artery technique after you have performed all techniques for all diaphragms (pelvic diaphragm, respiratory abdominal diaphragm, thoracic inlet, and cranial diaphragm) bilateral. This is an excellent technique for use with TOS (Thoracic outlet) and RSD (Reflex Sympathetic Dystrophy). Whenever there is compression of the brachial plexus within the costoclavicular joint space there is likely to be compromise of arterial flow of the subclavian artery. This technique can be preceded by the Advanced Strain /Counterstrain technique for the subclavius muscle. To decompress the subclavian artery 100%, first follow this sequence of Jones Strain and Counterstrain technique to open the costoclavicular joint: anterior first thoracic, anterior seventh and eighth cervical, elevated first rib, lateral cervicals (middle scalenes which elevate the first rib), anterior and posterior acromioclavicular joint. The client may have the following symtomatology: cyanosis or mild blueness of the finger nails, perspiration of the hand and/or clamminess, pain and or paresthesia of the extremity, headaches, dizziness and lightheadedness, vertigo. Remember, there is tension of the subclavian artery towards the vertebral arteries and into the basilar system.

CHAPTER 16

ADVANCED STRAIN AND COUNTERSTRAIN FOR ARTERIES
Arteries to the Urogenital Tissues

Art/UG1: Arteries of Capsule of Kidney
(Netter's plate #315–326)
(Bilateral)

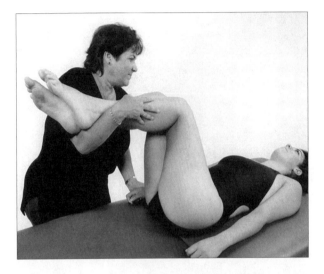

TENDER POINT

2 inches lateral to the 12th rib articulation (costovertebral joint) and 1 inch caudal.

TREATMENT

- Supine.
- Bilateral hip flexion to 90 degrees.
- Bilateral knee flexion to 110 degrees.
- Bring both knees to the ipsilateral side 20 degrees.
- Arm pull of the ipsilateral arm (longitudinal traction) in neutral with 10 lbs. force.

GOAL

Release of the smooth muscles of the arteries of capsule of kidney.

INTEGRATIVE MANUAL THERAPY™

PLEASE PERFORM THE ARTERIES OF CAPSULE OF KIDNEY TECHNIQUE AFTER YOU HAVE PERFORMED ALL OF THE TECHNIQUES FOR ALL OF THE DIAPHRAGMS (PELVIC DIAPHRAGM, RESPIRATORY ABDOMINAL DIAPHRAGM, THORACIC INLET, AND CRANIAL DIAPHRAGM) BILATERAL. Often there are problems secondary to blood pressure, cardiac and pericardial pressure, kidney and liver tensions, which affect the capsules of the kidneys because of arterial blood flow complications. The results of this technique may be improved kidney function, observed as: decreases in urinary incontinence, less urinary urgency, less burning during urination, and more. The most measurable change resulting from this technique will be increased in low thoracic and upper lumbar ranges of motion, with decreases in back pain.

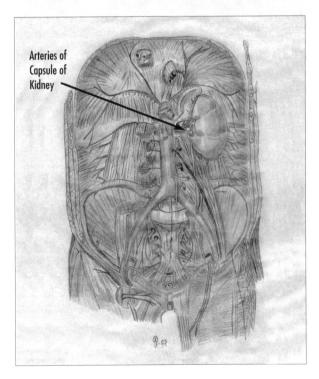

Arteries of Capsule of Kidney

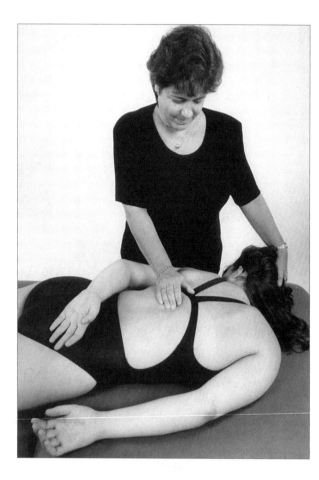

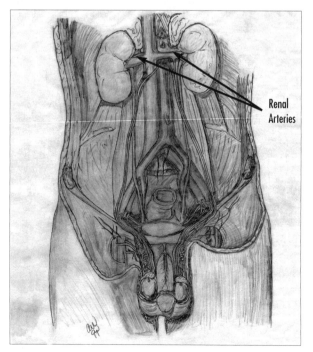

Renal
Arteries

Art/UG2: Renal Artery

(Netter's plate #247, 315–326)
(Bilateral)

TENDER POINT

Under anterior aspect of the 9th rib, 3 inches
lateral from sternum border.

TREATMENT

- Prone.
- Cervical rotation to the ipsilateral side to 60
  degrees.
- Cervical side bending to the ipsilateral side to
  30 degrees.
- Ipsilateral shoulder girdle depression to 15
  degrees (compress from the superior aspect
  of acromion).
- Dorsal aspect of ipsilateral hand rests on
  contralateral SI joint.
- Trunk side bending to the ipsilateral side 15
  degrees.
- Compress T10 spinous process in a lateral
  glide towards the ipsilateral side.
- Compress the ipsilateral 9th rib angle medial
  with over-pressure of 1 lb. force.

GOAL

Release of the smooth muscles of the renal
artery.

INTEGRATIVE MANUAL THERAPY™

PLEASE PERFORM THE RENAL ARTERY TECH-
NIQUE AFTER YOU HAVE PERFORMED ALL OF
THE TECHNIQUES FOR ALL OF THE
DIAPHRAGMS (PELVIC DIAPHRAGM, RESPIRA-
TORY ABDOMINAL DIAPHRAGM, THORACIC
INLET, AND CRANIAL DIAPHRAGM) BILATERAL.
Often there is tissue tightness of the low back because
of hypertonicity of the renal artery musculature. The
body protects arteries because of the major function of
arteries, and because of the fragile and delicate nature
of the membrane of the blood vessel. The low back
tension will occur because the muscle spasm and the
fascial tightness is present to protect the renal artery.

Therefore there will be increased lumbar spine ranges of motion after this technique is performed. Occasionally, these restrictions of the renal artery inhibit successful mobilization of the tissue surrounding the kidney, which is stuck and requires Visceral Manipulation (Barral).

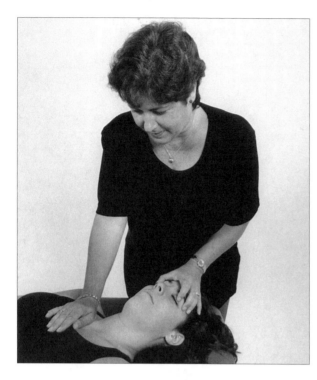

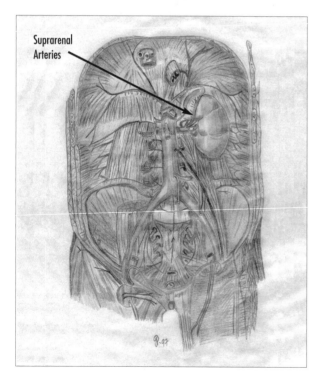

Suprarenal
Arteries

Art/UG3: Suprarenal Artery

(Netter's plate #315–326)
(Bilateral)

TENDER POINT

Posterior sternal notch, slightly medial to the sternoclavicular joint.

TREATMENT

- Supine.
- Hips and knees bent.
- Patient's ipsilateral hand reaches to rest under the ipsilateral ischial tuberosity.
- Trunk side bending to the ipsilateral side 5–10 degrees.
- Ipsilateral shoulder girdle depression 15 degrees.
- Cervical side bending to the ipsilateral side 5–10 degrees.
- Compress over the ipsilateral sternoclavicular joint in an inferior direction.

GOAL

Release of the smooth muscles of the suprarenal artery.

INTEGRATIVE MANUAL THERAPY™

PLEASE PERFORM THE SUPRARENAL ARTERY TECHNIQUE AFTER YOU HAVE PERFORMED ALL OF THE TECHNIQUES FOR ALL OF THE DIAPHRAGMS (PELVIC DIAPHRAGM, RESPIRATORY ABDOMINAL DIAPHRAGM, THORACIC INLET, AND CRANIAL DIAPHRAGM) . This technique often changes a lot more signs and symptoms than anticipated by the practitioner. The low thoracic and upper lumbar soft tissue often contracts around the suprarenal artery for protection of the artery. There will be increases in all ranges of thoracolumbar spinal movements, and a decrease in the hypertonicity of the respiratory abdominal diaphragm, with increased rib excursion with respiration. Mostly, these arteries are often in a state of hypertonicity secondary to adrenal gland energies that are stress related. There may be a change in the behavior of the person treated, with an increased threshold to stress.

Art/UGF/M1: Testicular/Ovarian Artery

(Netter's plate #247, 350, 365, 375–380)
(Bilateral)

TENDER POINT

Lateral to the pubic tubercle

TREATMENT

- Supine.
- Hips and knees are flexed, with feet on the bed.
- Knees are hyperflexed, so the feet are touching the buttock.
- "Inflare" the ipsilateral ASIS (compress the ilium towards medial rotation).
- Compress the ilium into anterior rotation.
- Bilateral tibial internal rotation (turn the feet inwards).

GOAL

Release of the smooth muscles of the testicular/ovarian artery.

INTEGRATIVE MANUAL THERAPY™

PLEASE PERFORM THE TESTICULAR/OVARIAN ARTERY TECHNIQUE AFTER YOU HAVE PERFORMED ALL OF THE TECHNIQUES FOR ALL OF THE DIAPHRAGMS (PELVIC DIAPHRAGM, RESPIRATORY ABDOMINAL DIAPHRAGM, THORACIC INLET, AND CRANIAL DIAPHRAGM) BILATERAL. Degeneration of the tissues of the testicles and ovaries is not rare, especially after infections, inflammation, surgeries, radiation and chemotherapy. This technique will restore circulation to the testicles and ovaries in many cases, evident by the change in tissue tension, and function.

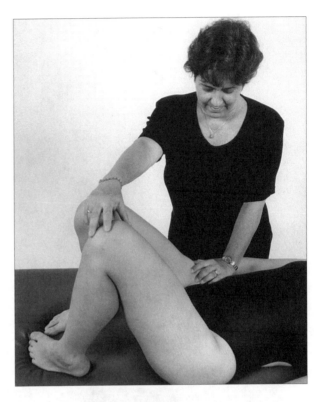

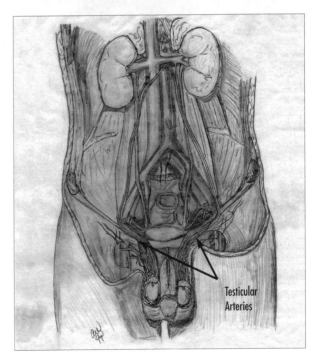

Testicular
Arteries

ADVANCED STRAIN AND COUNTERSTRAIN FOR ARTERIES
Arteries to the Spine

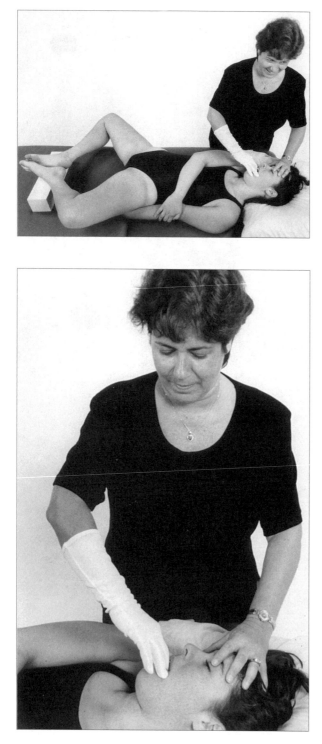

Art/Spine1: Anterior and Posterior Spinal Arteries
(Netter's plate #52, 53, 156, 158)
(Unilateral)

TENDER POINT

Base of occiput, 1 cm to left of midline.

TREATMENT

- (Intra-oral technique.)
- Supine.
- Therapist stands on the right side of the patient.
- Hips are flexed so that knees are both flexed to 120 degrees.
- The feet are placed on a 3 inch high towel roll or block (the feet are therefore 3 inches off the bed).
- Knees into full abduction.
- The soles of the feet touch each other.
- Trunk side bending to the left 15 degrees.
- Cervical flexion of 10 degrees. (Head place on a pillow)
- Cervical rotation to the right 15 degrees.
- Cervical side bending to the right 15 degrees.
- Patient's left hand reaches to rest on the left ischial tuberosity.
- Patient's right hand reaches to rest on the left forearm.
- Therapist's finger (of the right hand) is placed on the middle 1/3 of the median sulcus of the tongue.
- Compress the tongue inferior and anterior.
- Therapist's left hand is placed (gently) on patient's closed eye lids. Therapist compresses eye balls with 1 gram of pressure in posterior and inferior directions.

GOAL

Release of the smooth muscles of the anterior and posterior spinal arteries.

INTEGRATIVE MANUAL THERAPY™

PLEASE PERFORM THE ANTERIOR AND POSTE-RIOR SPINAL ARTERIES TECHNIQUE AFTER YOU HAVE PERFORMED ALL OF THE TECHNIQUES FOR ALL OF THE DIAPHRAGMS (PELVIC DIAPHRAGM, RESPIRATORY ABDOMI-NAL DIAPHRAGM, THORACIC INLET, AND CRA-NIAL DIAPHRAGM) BILATERAL. An interesting and remarkable phenomenon occurs with this technique: excellent elongation of the spine. This appears to be secondary to the elimination of the hypertonicity of the spinal arteries, which then results in elimination of neural contraction around the arteries which initially occurred to protect the compromised vascular tissues. Approximately 15% of spinal cord fibrosis will disappear immediately after utilization of this technique. Spinal pain is often decreased, but even more there are changes of all of the soft tissues and viscera which are innervated from the spinal cord. When there is hypertonicity of the muscles of the spinal arteries, there is a shortening of the spinal column in order to prevent further traction tension on the arteries. The vertebrae compression, which is the cause of the shortening of the spinal column, causes compromise and compression of the spinal nerve roots. This compression of the nerve roots can cause hypertonicity of all musculature in the body, and hypertonicity of visceral muscles, as well as spasm of the blood vessel muscles which are innervated by the continuation of these nerve roots. Documented cases of spinal cord injured patients, paraplegic and quadraparesis, are some of the case histories which indicate that this technique can be used with all spinal and back patients.

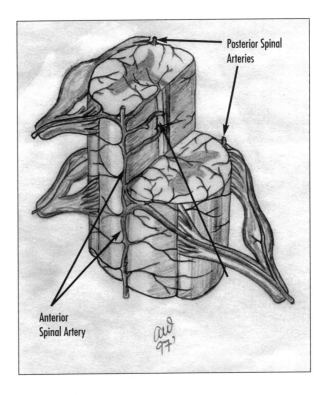

Posterior Spinal Arteries

Anterior Spinal Artery

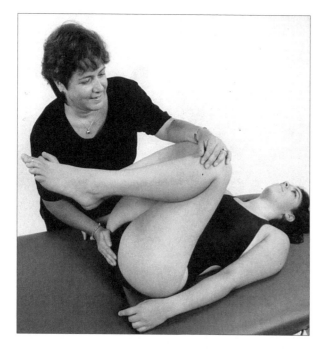

Art/Spine2: Middle Sacral Artery (Sacro-Coccyx Artery)

(Netter's plate #157, 247, 373)
(Bilateral)

TENDER POINT

Distal portion of the coccyx.

TREATMENT

- Supine.
- Bilateral knee flexion to the chest.
- Compress with over-pressure on both ischial tuberosities in a medial direction (squeeze the ischial tuberosities together).
- Compress the ipsilateral ischial tuberosity in an anterior direction.

GOAL

Release of the smooth muscles of the sacral-coccyx artery.

INTEGRATIVE MANUAL THERAPY™

PLEASE PERFORM THE MIDDLE SACRAL ARTERY TECHNIQUE AFTER YOU HAVE PER-FORMED ALL OF THE TECHNIQUES FOR ALL OF THE DIAPHRAGMS (PELVIC DIAPHRAGM, RESPI-RATORY ABDOMINAL DIAPHRAGM, THORACIC INLET, AND CRANIAL DIAPHRAGM) BILATERAL. Occasionally there will be a remarkable decrease in buttocks and tail-bone pain. Hemorrhoids may be affected. Women after episiotomies and difficult deliv-ery may describe marked decrease in pelvic discomfort after this technique. Occasionally there is significant hypertonicity and fascial dysfunction of the pelvic floor soft tissue, which has contracted in order to protect this artery. In these cases, there will be an exceptional improvement of function with this approach.

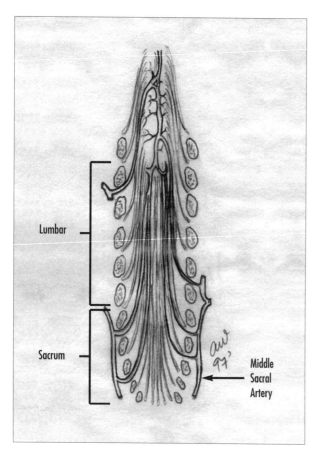

Lumbar

Sacrum

Middle Sacral Artery

Art/Spine3: Pial Arterial Plexus (Accessory Meningeal Artery)

(Netter's plate #158)
(Bilateral)
(Multiple spinal segments)

TENDER POINT

On the posterior aspect of the spinous process of each segment treated.

TREATMENT

- Supine.
- "Lift" the vertebral segment treated via compression anterior from the tip of the spinous process towards the ceiling with a 5 gram force.
- Then compress the spinous process superior, with 5 grams force.
- Maintain the compression and place the spine into flexion down/up the spinal kinetic chain to flex the vertebral segment being treated.

GOAL

Release of the smooth muscles of the accessory meningeal artery.

INTEGRATIVE MANUAL THERAPY™

PLEASE PERFORM THE PIAL ARTERIAL PLEXUS TECHNIQUE AFTER YOU HAVE PERFORMED ALL OF THE TECHNIQUES FOR ALL OF THE DIAPHRAGMS (PELVIC DIAPHRAGM, RESPIRATORY ABDOMINAL DIAPHRAGM, THORACIC INLET, AND CRANIAL DIAPHRAGM) BILATERAL. This technique can be used for all spinal patients, whether for back pain relief or spinal cord injury. Often there is low grade arachnoiditis after trauma, after surgery, after disease. This technique is excellent for treatment of arachnoiditis. Occasionally spinal cord fibrosis is perceived when there is really contraction of the spinal cord around the meningeal artery. This technique can be performed prior to cranial therapy, and prior to neurofascial release (Weiselfish-Giammatteo).

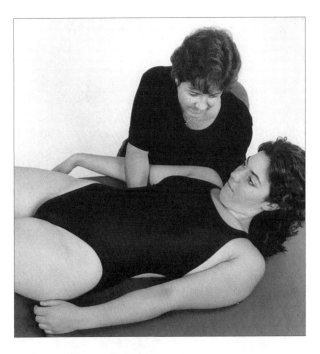

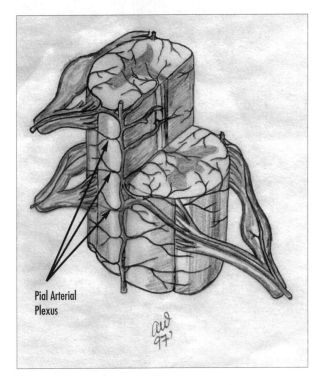

Pial Arterial Plexus

CHAPTER 18

ADVANCED STRAIN AND COUNTERSTRAIN FOR VEINS
Lower Extremities

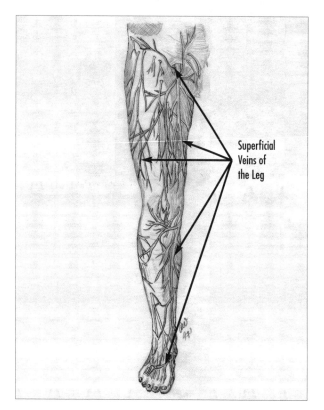

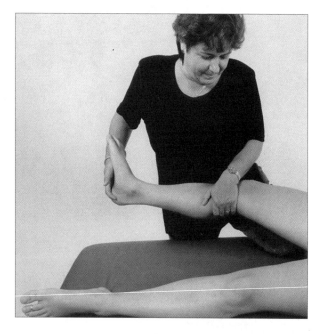

Superficial
Veins of
the Leg

Vein/LE1: Superficial Veins of the Lower Limbs

(Netter's plate #512, 513)
(Bilateral)

TENDER POINT

Popliteal fossa, 1 inch lateral to mid-line. Press deep into fossa and then compress lateral.

TREATMENT

- Supine.
- Hip flexion to 20 degrees.
- Hip abduction to 20 degrees.
- Hip external rotation to 5 degrees.
- Knee flexion to 5 degrees.
- Push on proximal tibial head for lateral glide with 5 lbs. of force.
- Dorsiflexion to 5 degrees.

GOAL

Release of the smooth muscles of the superficial veins of the lower limbs.

INTEGRATIVE MANUAL THERAPY™

All treatment of myofascial dysfunction and burn or scar tissue will be facilitated with this technique.

CHAPTER 19

ADVANCED STRAIN AND COUNTERSTRAIN FOR VEINS
Upper Extremities

Vein/UE1: Superficial Veins of the Arms
(Netter's plate #410, 452, 453)
(Bilateral)

TENDER POINT

In axilla, on the humeral head, mid-axillary line.

TREATMENT

- Supine.
- Caudal compression of the humeral head with 1 lb. of force.
- Horizontal adduction of arm to 50 degrees.
- Place hand over (anterior to) junction of the arm/thoracic cage.
- Compress in a posterior direction(anterior to posterior). Cover a large surface area with 1 lb. of force.
- Elbow is straight.

GOAL

Release of the smooth muscles of the superficial veins of the arms.

INTEGRATIVE MANUAL THERAPY™

This technique will be an excellent adjunct with manual therapy for all vascular and somatic dysfunctions of the upper extremity, necessary for burn therapy, treatment of myofascial dysfunction and scar tissue.

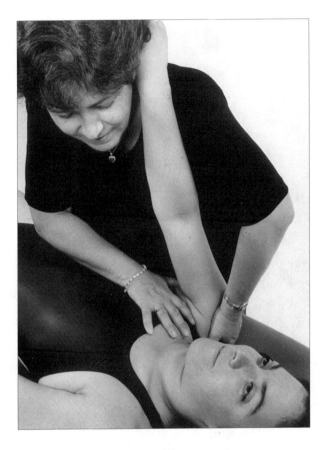

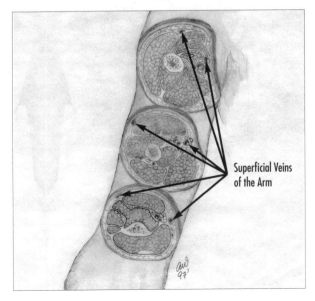

Superficial Veins of the Arm

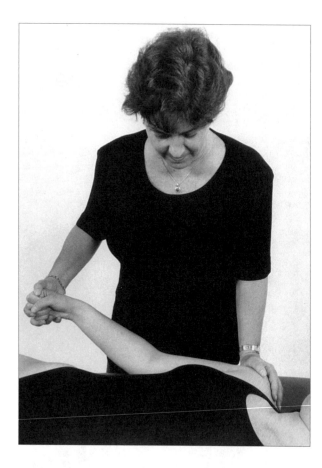

Vein/UE2: Superficial Veins of the Shoulder
(Netter's plate #410, 452)
(Bilateral)

TENDER POINT

On lower inner arm, in soft tissue, one (1) inch above nipple line.

TREATMENT

- Supine.
- Shoulder joint compression. Approximate the humeral head towards the glenoid fossa.
- Shoulder joint otherwise rests in anatomic neutral.
- Elbow flexion to 15 degrees.
- Pronation of forearm to 15 degrees.
- Wrist flexion to 5 degrees.
- Ulnar deviation to 5 degrees.
- Fingers flexed into a fist.

GOAL

Release of the smooth muscles of the superficial veins of the shoulder.

INTEGRATIVE MANUAL THERAPY™

Swelling of the glenohumeral joint after trauma will be alleviated quickly if this technique is performed during the acute phase.

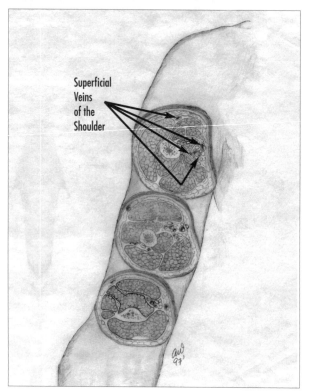

Superficial Veins of the Shoulder

CHAPTER 20

ADVANCED STRAIN AND COUNTERSTRAIN FOR VEINS
Cranial and Cervical Veins

Vein/Cranial 1: Superficial Cerebral Veins
(Netter's plate #96)
(Bilateral)

TENDER POINT

The junction of the occipitomastoid suture and
the suboccipital soft tissue. Compress superior
into the soft tissue.

TREATMENT

- Supine.
- Lengthen the neck on the side of the Tender
  Point with longitudinal stretching of the mas-
  toid process (occiput and temporal) away.
- Fixate the shoulder girdle.
- Gently push the mastoid process anterior
  with 5 grams of force.

GOAL

Release of the smooth muscles of the superficial
cerebral veins.

INTEGRATIVE MANUAL THERAPY™

PLEASE PERFORM THE SUPERFICIAL CERE-
BRAL VEIN TECHNIQUE AFTER YOU HAVE PER-
FORMED ALL OF THE TECHNIQUES FOR ALL OF
THE DIAPHRAGMS (PELVIC DIAPHRAGM, RESPI-
RATORY ABDOMINAL DIAPHRAGM, THORACIC
INLET, AND CRANIAL DIAPHRAGM) BILATERAL.
Often this technique will eliminate or decrease scalp
itchiness, dandruff, and may partially contribute to
increased hair growth. The scalp is an area of "toxin
attraction." This technique may facilitate detoxification
of the scalp. Scars after surgery and trauma will heal
faster, and there will be less likelihood for dysfunction
to occur secondary to fascial tightness when this technique is used in acute stages after surgery and trauma.

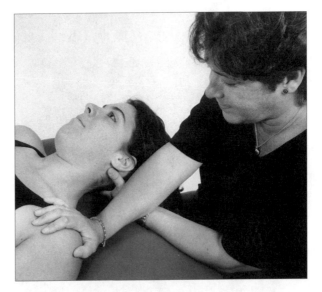

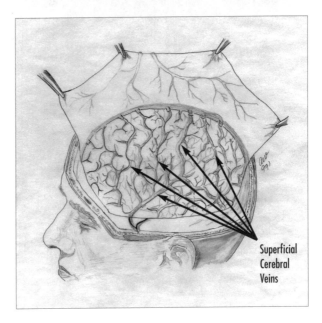

Superficial
Cerebral
Veins

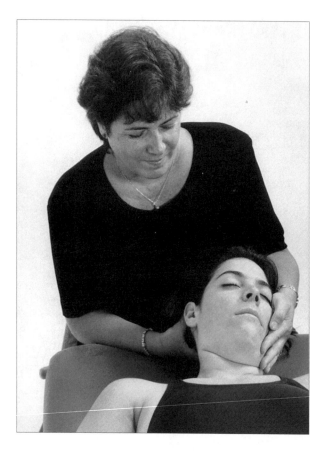

Vein/Cranial 2: Superficial Veins of the Head
(Netter's plate #17)
(bilateral)

TENDER POINT

On the cheek, just inferior to zygoma, 3 inches
anterior to the meatus.

TREATMENT

- Supine.
- Forceful traction of the cheek soft tissue inferior, while the hand is over the zygoma,
  cheek and mandible.
- Neck flexion to 20 degrees.
- Neck rotation to the ipsilateral side to 30
  degrees.

GOAL

Release of the smooth muscles of the superficial
veins of the head.

INTEGRATIVE MANUAL THERAPY™

PLEASE PERFORM THE SUPERFICIAL VEINS OF
THE HEAD TECHNIQUE AFTER YOU HAVE PER-
FORMED ALL OF THE TECHNIQUES FOR ALL OF
THE DIAPHRAGMS (PELVIC DIAPHRAGM, RESPI-
RATORY ABDOMINAL DIAPHRAGM, THORACIC
INLET, AND CRANIAL DIAPHRAGM) BILATERAL.
This technique is generally effective to decrease intra-
cranial edema in acute head trauma. It is less effective
in chronic cerebral swelling.

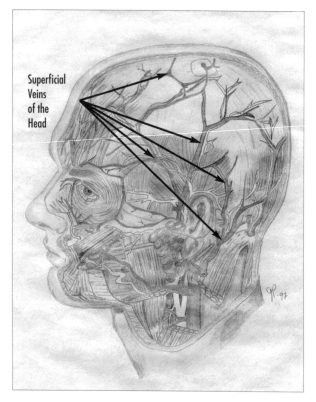

Superficial
Veins
of the
Head

Vein/Cranial 3: Superficial Veins of the Neck
(Netter's plate #26)
(Bilateral)

TENDER POINT

Lower sternal notch, penetrate posterior from the sternal notch into the soft tissue, 1 finger breadth lateral to side of tender point.

TREATMENT

- Supine.
- Neck flexion to 20 degrees.
- Neck rotation to the ipsilateral side to 30 degrees.
- Neck side bending to the ipsilateral side to 20 degrees.
- Place a hand behind (posterior to) neck.
- Compress posterior to anterior into the sternal notch from C5 and C6 vertebrae.

GOAL

Release of the smooth muscles of the superficial veins of the neck.

INTEGRATIVE MANUAL THERAPY™

PLEASE PERFORM THE SUPERFICIAL VEINS OF THE NECK TECHNIQUE AFTER YOU HAVE PERFORMED ALL OF THE TECHNIQUES FOR ALL OF THE DIAPHRAGMS (PELVIC DIAPHRAGM, RESPIRATORY ABDOMINAL DIAPHRAGM, THORACIC INLET, AND CRANIAL DIAPHRAGM) BILATERAL. There is an extensive network of superficial veins of the neck, which is partially because of the vast number of lymph nodes at the lateral neck. The veins are easily congested, especially secondary to protective muscle spasm of the anterior cervical muscles and the hyoid musculature. These muscle are hypertonic when the person represses expression of emotions and thoughts. Therefore, it is always beneficial to precede this technique with Jones Strain and Counterstrain for all of the anterior cervical techniques. This Advanced Strain/Counterstrain technique for the superficial veins of the neck is excellent to alleviate swelling of the 'double chin' sort, and may improve speech and swallowing.

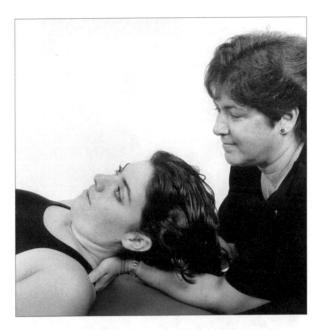

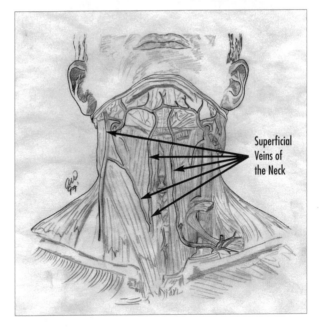

Superficial Veins of the Neck

CHAPTER 21

ADVANCED STRAIN AND COUNTERSTRAIN FOR VEINS
Cardiopulmonary Veins

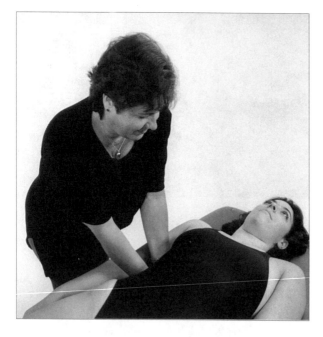

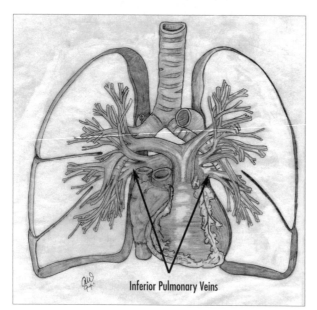

Inferior Pulmonary Veins

Vein/Cardio1: Alveolar—Inferior Pulmonary Veins
(Netter's plate #194, 195)
(Bilateral)
(Multiple levels)

TENDER POINT

On the lung, at the rib angle, on each of the 12 ribs. Press onto lungs.

TREATMENT

- Supine (not prone: for postural drainage)
- Compress over the Tender Point (on the rib angle) in anterior and medial directions with 5 grams of force.
- Push the rib medial, compressing the costovertebral joint.
- Compress the medial aspect of the rib in an anterior direction with 5 grams of force. (There are 12 techniques, for each right and left Lung.)

GOAL

Release of the smooth muscles of the inferior alveolar vein. Improve respiratory function.

INTEGRATIVE MANUAL THERAPY™

Be prepared for significant changes with this technique: intra-thoracic edema will subside, and all pulmonary disorders which are partially the result of the edema will improve. Coughing, sleep apnea, sneezing, hiccuping, burping, choking and other behaviors may decrease in intensity and frequency. All pulmonary disorders, including asthma, emphysema, atelectasis, bronchial disorders, and the like may improve.

Vein/Cardio2: Alveolar— Superior Pulmonary Vein

(Netter's plate #194, 195)
(Bilateral)
(Multiple levels)

TENDER POINT

On the lung, at the inner (medial) aspect of the rib angle, on each of the 12 ribs.

TREATMENT

- Supine (not prone).
- Push rib lateral from the Tender Point (which is on the medial aspect of the rib angle) with 5 grams of force.
- Compress the total lung, of the side treated, anterior to posterior with 5 grams of pressure.
  (Push the total lung with the pressure from this rib.)
  (There are 12 techniques each on right and left lung.)

GOAL

Release of the smooth muscles of the posterior superior alveolar vein. Improve respiratory function.

INTEGRATIVE MANUAL THERAPY™

Be prepared for significant changes with this technique: intra-thoracic edema will subside, and all pulmonary disorders which are partially the result of the edema will improve. Coughing, sleep apnea, sneezing, hiccuping, burping, choking and other behaviors may decrease in intensity and frequency. All pulmonary disorders, including asthma, emphysema, atelectasis, bronchial disorders, and the like may improve.

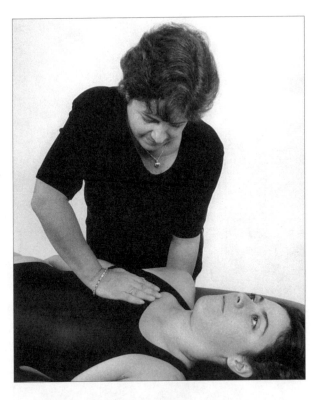

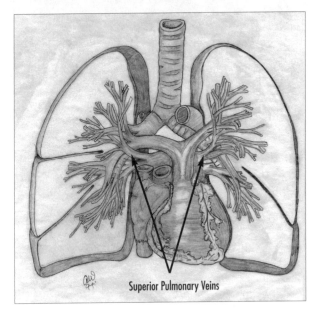

Superior Pulmonary Veins

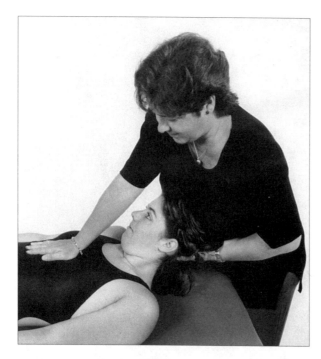

Vein/Cardio3: Superficial Veins of the Trunk
(Netter's plate #239)
(Bilateral)

TENDER POINT

Superior to sternoxiphoid junction. Lateral from midline 1 finger breadth to side of Tender Point.

TREATMENT

- Supine.
- Compress over the Tender Point in inferior and posterior and lateral directions with 5 grams of force.
- Neck flexion to 50 degrees.
- Neck rotation to 20 degrees to the ipsilateral side.

GOAL

Release of the smooth muscles of the superficial veins of the trunk. Improve respiratory function.

INTEGRATIVE MANUAL THERAPY™

Be prepared for significant changes with this technique: intra-thoracic edema will subside, and all pulmonary disorders which are partially the result of the edema will improve. Coughing, sleep apnea, sneezing, hiccuping, burping, choking and other behaviors may decrease in intensity and frequency. All pulmonary disorders, including asthma, emphysema, atelectasis, bronchial disorders, and the like may improve.

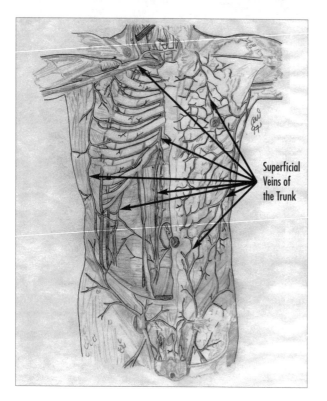

Superficial Veins of the Trunk

Vein/Cardio4: Inferior Vena Cava

(Netter's plate #202, 203, 208, 217)
(Unilateral)

TENDER POINT

Mid-line of the sternum at the level of the 6th rib.

TREATMENT

- Supine/Sitting.
- Therapist stands to the right of the patient.
- Bilateral transverse processes of T8 are compressed medial.
- Left knee bent/normal sitting position.
- Right ankle is placed onto left knee.
- Compress posterior, superior, and lateral direction, 1 inch lateral to the right 8th intracostal cartilage, with 5–10 grams of pressure.

INTEGRATIVE MANUAL THERAPY™

PLEASE PERFORM THE INFERIOR VENA CAVA TECHNIQUE AFTER YOU HAVE PERFORMED ALL OF THE TECHNIQUES FOR ALL OF THE DIAPHRAGMS (PELVIC DIAPHRAGM, RESPIRATORY ABDOMINAL DIAPHRAGM, THORACIC INLET, AND CRANIAL DIAPHRAGM) BILATERAL. Both Advanced Strain and Counterstrain techniques for the Superior and the Inferior Vena Cava should always be performed together, and they should be performed before too many arterial techniques are performed. Possibly use this technique before all arterial (aorta technique included) techniques are performed, to get into the correct 'habit.' Treatment reactions could otherwise occur, due to improved vascular output without sufficient drainage of fluid (H_2O) from the interstitium via the venous system. The Superior and Inferior Vena Cava techniques are excellent for all of the following: regional and total body edema; lymphedema; lipedema; all fibromyalgia-like syndromes; all scars and other connective tissue problems of hypertrophy and hyperplasia; all respiratory disorders; all cardiopulmonary and cardiovascular disorders; all brain and spinal cord dysfunction, whether mild or severe, chronic or acute. There are no contraindications for these techniques.

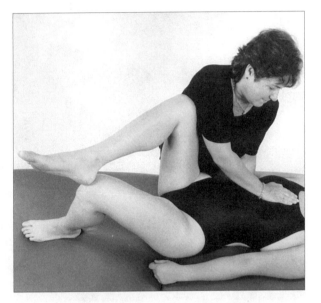

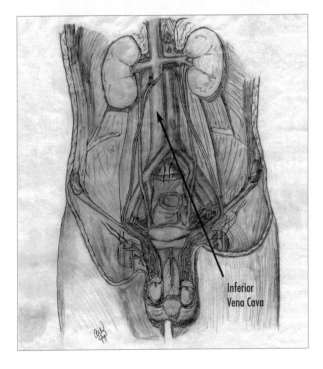

Inferior Vena Cava

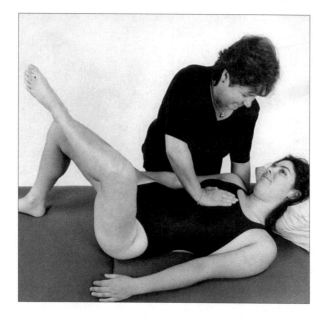

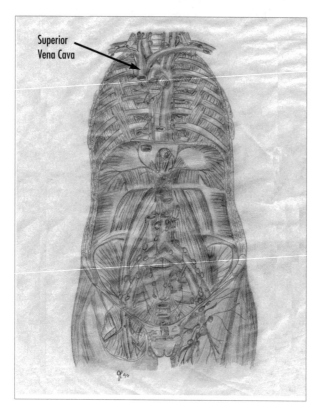

Superior
Vena Cava

Vein/Cardio5: Superior Vena Cava

(Netter's plate #201, 202, 203, 208, 217)
(Unilateral)

TENDER POINT

Mid-line of the sternum at the level of the 3rd rib.

TREATMENT

- Supine/Sitting
- Therapist stands to the right of the patient.
- Bilateral transverse processes of T5 are compressed medial.
- Right knee bent/normal sitting position.
- Left ankle placed onto right knee.
- Trunk side bending to the right 10-15 degrees.
- Cervical flexion 30 degrees.
- Cervical rotation to the right 10 degrees.
- Cervical side bending to the right 5 degrees.
- Compress in posterior, superior and lateral directions, 1 inch lateral to the right 8th intracostal cartilage with 5-10 grams of pressure.

GOAL

Release of the smooth muscles of the superior vena cava.

INTEGRATIVE MANUAL THERAPY™

PLEASE PERFORM THE SUPERIOR VENA CAVA TECHNIQUE AFTER YOU HAVE PERFORMED ALL OF THE TECHNIQUES FOR ALL OF THE DIAPHRAGMS (PELVIC DIAPHRAGM, RESPIRATORY ABDOMINAL DIAPHRAGM, THORACIC INLET, AND CRANIAL DIAPHRAGM) BILATERAL. Both Advanced Strain and Counterstrain techniques for the Superior and the Inferior Vena Cava should always be performed together, and they should be performed before too many arterial techniques are performed. Possibly use this technique before all arterial (aorta

technique included) techniques are performed, to
get into the correct 'habit.' Treatment reactions could
otherwise occur, due to improved vascular output without sufficient drainage of fluid (H_2O) from the interstitium via the venous system. The Superior and Inferior
Vena Cava techniques are excellent for all of the following: regional and total body edema; lymphedema;
lipedema; all fibromyalgia-like syndromes; all scars
and other connective tissue problems of hypertrophy
and hyperplasia; all respiratory disorders; all cardiopulmonary and cardiovascular disorders; all brain
and spinal cord dysfunction, whether mild or severe,
chronic or acute. There are no contraindications for
these techniques.

CHAPTER 22

ADVANCED STRAIN AND COUNTERSTRAIN FOR VEINS
Visceral Veins

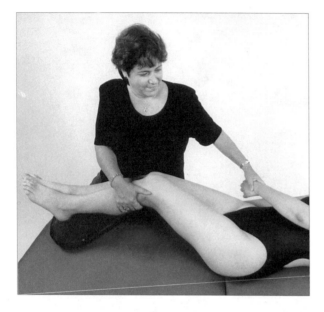

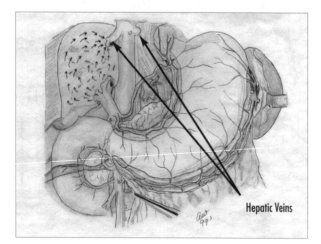

Hepatic Veins

Vein/Org1: Hepatic Vein
(Netter's plate #294)
(Unilateral)

TENDER POINT

On the lingula (tongue) of the liver, at the superior/anterior aspect, just left of the falciform ligament.

TREATMENT

- Supine.
- Flex both hips 30 degrees.
- Flex both knees 20 degrees.
- Rotate the knees (bring the knees lateral) to the right side 10 degrees.
- The left hand is pulled towards the lower right rib cage.

GOAL

To eliminate the hypertonicity of the muscles of the portal vein.

INTEGRATIVE MANUAL THERAPY™

This technique should be used together with the technique for the Portal Vein. Often this technique can be used after the Advanced Strain/Counterstrain technique for the liver, followed by all of the renal procedures, including: hilum of kidneys, renal arteries, ureters, bladder and urethra. Typically there will be an improvement in elimination. Occasionally blood pressure will be normalized. Fibromyalgia-like syndromes can often be improved because of the changes in detoxification by the liver.

Vein/Org2: Portal Vein

(Netter's plate #294-298)
(Unilateral)

TENDER POINT

On the inferior aspect of the liver, two inches medial from the lateral border of the right rib cage.

TREATMENT

- Supine.
- Flex both hips to 90 degrees.
- Flex both knees to 120 degrees.
- Rotate the knees (bring the knees to the right) 20 degrees.
- Pull on the right hand inferior for longitudinal traction of the right arm.

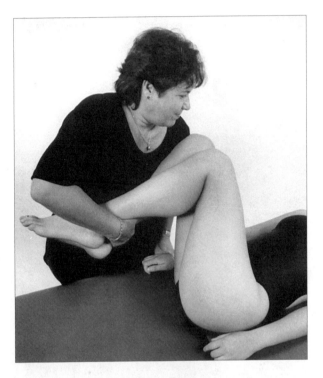

GOAL

To eliminate the hypertonicity of the muscles of the portal vein.

INTEGRATIVE MANUAL THERAPY™

This technique should be used together with the technique for the hepatic vein. Often this technique can be used after the Advanced Strain/Counterstrain technique for the liver, followed by all of the renal procedures, including: hilum of kidneys, renal arteries, ureters, bladder and urethra. Typically there will be an improvement in elimination. Occasionally blood pressure will be normalized. Fibromyalgia-like syndromes can often be improved because of the changes in detoxification by the liver.

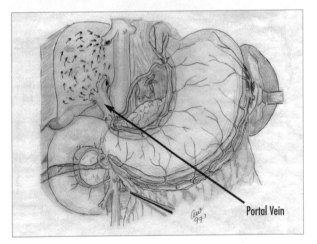

Portal Vein

CHAPTER 23

ADVANCED STRAIN AND COUNTERSTRAIN FOR VEINS
Spinal Veins

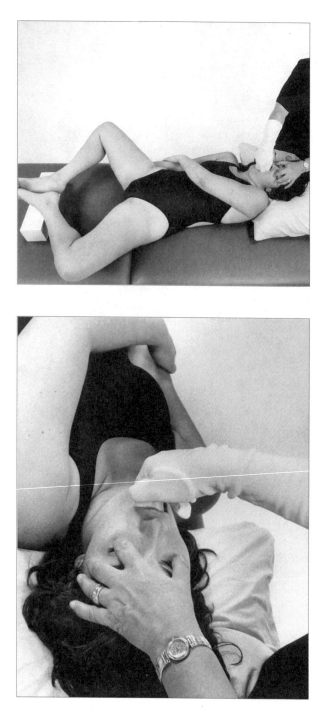

Vein/Spine1: Anterior and Posterior Spinal Veins
(Netter's plate #52, 53, 55, 156, 159)
(Unilateral)

TENDER POINT

Base of occiput, 1 cm to right of midline.

TREATMENT

(Intra-oral technique.)
- Supine.
- Therapist stands to the right side of the patient.
- Knees bent to 120 degrees.
- Feet are placed on a 3 inch towel roll or block.
- Knees in full abduction
- Soles of the feet touch each other.
- Trunk side bending to the right 15 degrees.
- Cervical flexion of 10 degrees. (Head place on a pillow)
- Cervical rotation to the left 20 degrees.
- Cervical side bending to the left 15 degrees.
- Patient's right hand reaches for the right ischial tuberosity and rests there.
- Patient's left hand reaches for and rests on the right forearm.
- Therapist's fingers are placed under the tongue. The therapist lifts tongue superior.
- Therapist's left hand is placed (gently) on patient's closed eye lids. Therapist compresses eye balls with 1 gram of pressure in posterior and superior directions.

GOAL

Release of the smooth muscles of the anterior and posterior spinal veins.

INTEGRATIVE MANUAL THERAPY™

PLEASE PERFORM THE ANTERIOR AND POSTE-
RIOR SPINAL VEINS TECHNIQUE AFTER YOU
HAVE PERFORMED ALL OF THE TECHNIQUES
FOR ALL OF THE DIAPHRAGMS (PELVIC
DIAPHRAGM, RESPIRATORY ABDOMINAL DI-
APHRAGM, THORACIC INLET, AND CRANIAL
DIAPHRAGM) BILATERAL. This technique can be
applied together with the technique for the spinal arteries. Whenever there is a history of arachnoiditis,
meningitis, encephalitis, and other inflammatory and
infectious problems of the spine and brain, this technique appears uniquely effective. This technique may
affect functional impairments of multiple sclerosis and
other central nervous system disorders with plaque
formation. There are no contraindications to this
technique.

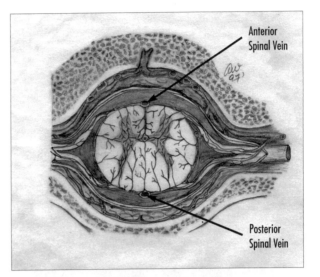

ADVANCED STRAIN AND COUNTERSTRAIN
Disc Therapy™

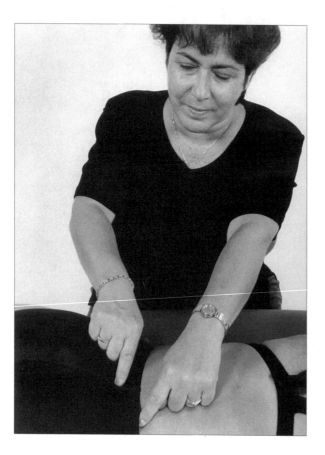

Advanced Strain and Counterstrain Technique for treatment of disc dysfunction provides evidence that the disc has contractile tissue which is innervated by the autonomic nervous system. Disc Therapy™ with Advanced Strain and Counterstrain Technique is simple to perform and the results are exceptional. Often the nerve root is impinged on the disc resulting in radiculopathy. Disc Therapy may mobilize the disc and radicular pain can be eliminated in this manner.

Image the disc similar to a radial tire. The annular fibers are the tire. There is also an inner lining. This inner lining of the disc appears to have contractile tissues which are also innervated by the autonomic nervous system. Both the annulus and the inner lining of the disc respond to Disc Therapy™. Further investigation into the histologic findings of the disc with electron microscopy studies are indicated, considering the response of the disc to Advanced Strain and Counterstrain Technique.

Phase One: Disc Therapy™ for the Annulus Fibrosis

Advanced Strain and Counterstrain Technique to eliminate the hypertonicity of the annulus fibrosis of the disc is as follows:

The client is in the prone position.

Step 1: Press on one of the transverse process of the vertebra which is superior to the involved disc. Press on either the right or left transverse process. Press from posterior to anterior and medial and inferior directions (1 lb. force).

Step 2: At the same time, press on the opposite transverse process of the vertebra inferior to the involved disc. This means, if the therapist presses on the right transverse process of the superior vertebra in Step One, the pressure will be on the left transverse process of the inferior vertebra. Press with 1 lb. force. Press from posterior to anterior and medial and superior directions.

Step 3 and 4:   Change the pressure to the opposite transverse processes. If the pressure was on the right superior transverse process and the left inferior transverse process, change the pressure to the left superior transverse process and the right inferior transverse process.

Step 5:   Determine the 'direction of ease.' Is Step One plus Step Two more or less resistant than Step Three and Four? Which 'set' of transverse processes is most mobile upon posterior to anterior pressure? Is there more or less tension when pressure is on the right superior transverse process together with the left inferior transverse process, as compared to the tension when pressure is on the left superior transverse process together with the right inferior transverse process? Choose the set of transverse processes which have less tension. Press posterior to anterior on these transverse processes. The inferior transverse process is pressed medial and superior. The superior transverse process is pressed medial and inferior.

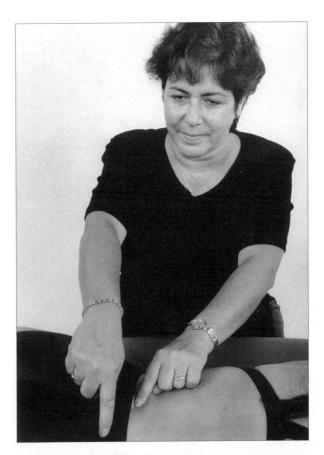

Step 6:   Maintain the compression on these two transverse processes for one minute, essentially bringing the two transverse processes closer together.

Step 7:   After one minute, change the pressure to the opposite transverse processes. If the pressure was on the right superior transverse process and the left inferior transverse process, change the pressure

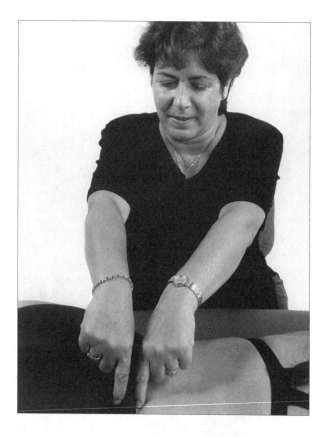

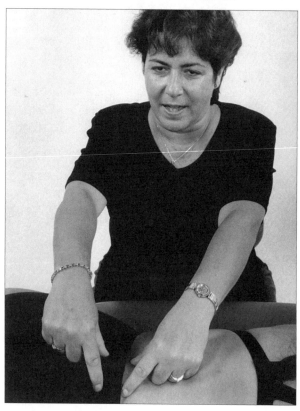

to the left superior transverse process and the right inferior transverse process.

Step 8: Maintain the posterior to anterior pressure for one (1) minute and continue to maintain the pressure for the duration of the De-Facilitated Fascial Release.

Phase Two: Disc Therapy™ for the Lining of the Disc

The client is prone.

Part I

Step 1: Pinch the superior and the inferior vertebrae of the involved disc at the same time. Grip at the spinous processes.

Step 2: Bring the two spinous processes closer together, towards each other. Essentially the superior vertebra is being extended, while the inferior is being flexed.

Step 3: Maintain the compression force which is bringing the two spinous process together for one minute.

Step 4: Maintain the compression for a DE-FACILITATED FASCIAL RELEASE™.

Part II

Step 1: Pinch the superior and the inferior vertebrae of the involved disc at the same time. Grip at the spinous processes.

Step 2: Bring the two spinous processes farther apart. Essentially the superior vertebra is being flexed, while the inferior is being extended.

Step 3: Maintain the tensile force which is bringing the two spinous process farther apart for one minute.

Step 4: Maintain the tension for a DE-FACILITATED FASCIAL RELEASE™.

Disc Therapy™ with Advanced Strain and Counterstrain is most effective after biomechanics of the pelvis, sacrum and spine have been restored.

This is best achieved with Muscle Energy 'Beyond' Technique developed by Weiselfish-Giammatteo, described in her book and videos and taught at (DCR) Dialogues In Contemporary Rehabilitation courses.

Disc Therapy for Knee Menisci, Temporomandibular Disc, and Other Menisci and Discs

Discs respond to Advanced Strain and Counterstrain with increased joint mobility, decreased muscle tone surrounding the joint, and increased ranges of motion.

Step 1. Place fingers at diagonal opposite ends of the disc: one finger proximal to the superior surface of one end of the disc; one finger distal to the inferior surface of the opposite end of the disc.

Step 2. Press on these diagonal opposite ends at the same time for one minute.

Step 3. Change finger placement to the ends of the disc which were not yet treated.

Step 4. Press on these diagonal opposite ends at the same time for one minute.

All discs and menisci can be treated in a similar manner. Be proximal to the disc and distal to the disc at the same time. Be at the anterior end of the disc and at the posterior end of the disc at the same time.

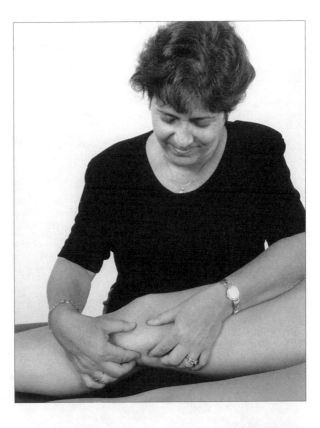

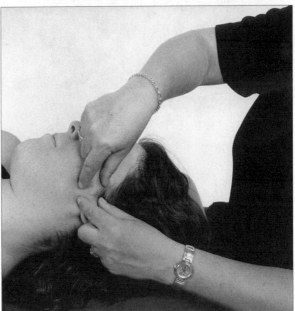

CHAPTER 25

ADVANCED STRAIN AND COUNTERSTRAIN
Tendon Release Therapy™

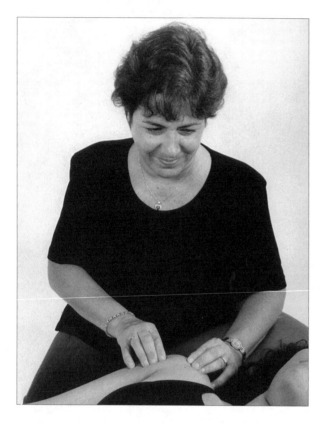

General Aspects of Advanced Strain and Counterstrain for Tendons

The tendons are apparently innervated by the autonomic nervous system, because functionally, they respond in a similar manner to smooth muscles. There is a passive contractile function, that is required for the stretch reflex of the proprioceptors, such as the Golgi Apparatus. The contractile tissues are longitudinal along the length of the tendon. When there is hypertonicity of a tendon, it presents as a rigidity of the tendon. There is a reduced capacity of elongation and contraction of the tendon fibers.

Treatment of tendons with Advanced Strain and Counterstrain is 1 minute because all innervated muscles require 1 minute for release of hypertonicity, as compared to 90 seconds release for voluntary nervous system innervated muscles. The process of *De-Facilitated Fascial Release*™ (for further explanation, refer to Chapter 4) works well with Tendon Release Therapy™.

Tendons of voluntary striated muscles are treated in a relatively simple manner with Advanced Strain and Counterstrain Technique, with excellent results. The distal and proximal ends of the tendon are pressed against the bone, pressing perpendicular through the fibers onto the bone. This pressure is at the insertion of the distal aspect of the tendon, when it inserts into the bone, and at the proximal aspect where the muscle fibers integrate with the tendon fibers. Maintaining this direct pressure of approximately 1 pound force, the distal and proximal ends of the tendon are pushed closer together. This compression is along the longitudinal length of the tendon fibers. The compression is maintained for 1 minute for release of hypertonicity of the tendon. There may remain fascial restrictions of the tendon, which may still require fascial release. The tendon responds well to *De-Facilitated Fascial Release*™.

Step-by-step Instructions for Tendon Release Therapy™

Step 1: Place the index finger (or the index finger plus the third finger) pad of the distal phalanx of the caudal hand over the place of insertion of the inferior end of the tendon.

Step 2: Place the index finger (or the index finger plus third finger) pad of the distal phalanx of the superior hand over the musculotendinous interface of the muscle/tendon, at the superior aspect of the tendon.

Step 3: Push on the tendon tissue with both hands (fingers) with 1 lb. force perpendicular onto the bone.

Step 4: Then compress the superior aspects and inferior aspects of the tendon together with 1 lb. force, bringing the proximal and distal ends of the tendon closer together.

Step 5: Maintain these (4) compressive forces for one minute for the Advanced Strain and Counterstrain.

Step 6: If fascial unwinding is perceived, maintain the (4) compressive forces during a *De-Facilitated Fascial Release*™.

Indications for Tendon Release Therapy™

There are essentially no contra-indications for Tendon Release Therapy™ when performed in this manner, unless there is a total rupture of the tendon. When there is a total rupture of the tendon, the technique will not be effective.

If there is a tear or rupture of the tendon, but there is a correction performed (surgical), the technique can be performed. Although not

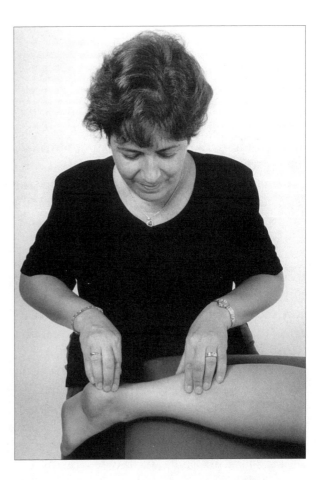

100% effective, the technique will give some results in decreased hypertonicity and rigidity of the tendon if the Tendon Release Therapy™ is performed immediately after surgery. There will be a facilitated healing of the tendonous injury.

Tendon Release Therapy™ is best performed after Strain and Counterstrain is performed to the muscle of the tendon. Often there is no remaining hypertonicity of the muscle, only of the tendon. In that case, Tendon Release Therapy™ can be performed without Strain and Counterstrain to the muscle.

After Tendon Release Therapy™ is performed, there may be some residual fascial dysfunction of the connective tissue of the tendon. This occurs most often when there are tears and scarring of the tendon. Then, after the Tendon Release Therapy™, a 3-Planar Fascial Fulcrum™ Technique (Myofascial Release, Weiselfish-Giammatteo) can be performed for optimal results, The Advanced Strain and Counterstrain Technique for the tendon (Tendon Release Therapy™) affects the hypertonicity of the tendon, resulting in a softening of the tendon and a decrease in the rigid presentation of that tendon. When De-Facilitated Fascial Release™ is performed immediately after the Tendon Release Therapy™, often the fascial dysfunction is corrected. When the scarring of the tendon (the fibrosis) is severe, there is often a need to perform the fascial release after the Tendon Release Therapy™.

Sequence of Strain and Counterstrain for Tendons

Step 1: Strain and Counterstrain for the muscle.

Step 2: De-Facilitated Fascial Release™ for the muscle.

Step 3: Tendon Release Therapy™ (Advanced Strain and Counterstrain).

Step 4: De-Facilitated Fascial Release™ for the tendon.

Step 5: Myofascial Release (3-Planar Fascial Fulcrum™) Tendon Technique.

Example of Advanced Strain and Counterstrain for Tendon Release: Achilles Tendon

TENDER POINT

At the insertion of the Achilles tendon

POSITION

Prone. A small towel roll is placed under the ankle, or the foot is off the edge of the bed, so that the foot and ankle are not in forced plantar flexion.

TREATMENT

- Place the index finger (or index finger plus the third finger) pad of the distal phalanx of the caudal hand over the place of insertion of the achilles tendon at the calcaneus.
- Place the index finger (or index finger plus third finger) pad of the distal phalanx of the superior hand over the musculotendinous interface of the gastrocnemius muscle with the achilles tendon, at the superior aspect of the tendon.
- Push the tissue with 1 lb. force perpendicular toward the tibia.
- Then compress the superior aspect and inferior aspect of the tendon together with about 1 lb. force, bringing the 2 ends of the tendon closer together.
- Maintain these compressive forces.

INTEGRATIVE MANUAL THERAPY™

Restoration of Dorsi-Flexion: Limitation of dorsi-flexion is a typical problem. There are many problems which result secondary to limited dorsi flexion. In mid-stance of the gait cycle, and during standing, the person needs to stand in anatomical zero (not plantar flexion, not dorsi flexion). When the person stands in plantar flexion (less than anatomical zero) there are extensor forces transcribed up the leg. These forces contribute to : shin splints; chondromalasia; genu recurvatum; extended sacral biomechanical problems; hypertonicity of extensor muscles. During mid-stance to toe off of stance phase, the tibia is supposed to glide anterior on talus approximately 10 degrees. Whenever there is less than 10 degrees dorsi flexion, mid-stance through toe-off is affected, and extensor forces are transcribed up the leg, causing biomechanical dysfunction, hypertonicity (muscle spasm), and fascial dysfunction.

To restore dorsiflexion, follow the following protocol:

Step 1: Strain and Counterstrain for the gastrocnemius, and a De-Facilitated Fascial Release™ for the gastrocnemius. (Jones Extended Ankle Technique)

Step 2: Muscle Belly Technique (Myofascial Release, Weiselfish-Giammatteo) for the gastrocnemius (if indicated by postural deviation of the gastrocnemius).

Step 3: Advanced Strain and Counterstrain (Tendon Release Therapy™) for the achilles tendon, and a De-Facilitated Fascial Release™ for the achilles tendon.

Step 4: 3-Planar Fascial Fulcrum™ (Myofascial Release) for the achilles tendon.

Step 5: When the sub-talar (talo-calcaneal) joint is still hypomobile, Strain and Counterstrain in the following sequence: Jones Medial Ankle Technique, Medial Calcaneal Technique, Lateral Ankle Technique, Lateral Calcaneal Technique.

Step 6: If there is any remaining hypomobility of the tibio-talar joint, manipulation of the tibio-talar joint (for intra-articular adhesions). (Muscle Energy and 'Beyond' Technique™, Weiselfish)

Step 7: If there is any remaining hypomobility of the sub-talar (talo-calcaneal) joint , manipulation of the sub-talar joint (for intra-articular adhesions). (Muscle Energy and 'Beyond' Technique™, Weiselfish)

Tendons which respond well to Tendon Release Therapy™

- Achilles Tendon
- Medial and Lateral Hamstrings Tendons
- Quadriceps Tendon
- Tibialis Anterior Tendon
- Tibialis Posterior Tendon
- Extensor Tendons of the Foot and Toes
- Flexor Tendons of the Foot and Toes
- Abductor Hallucis
- Adductor Tendons of the Hip
- Rotator Cuff Tendons: Supraspinatus, Infraspinatus, Subscapularis
- Latissimus Dorsi
- Biceps Tendons (Short Head and Long Head)
- Triceps Tendon
- Coracobrachialis Tendon
- Brachioradialis Tendon
- Wrist Flexor Tendons
- Wrist Extensor Tendons
- Finger Flexor Tendons
- Finger Extensor Tendons
- Abductor Pollicis Tendon
- Flexor Pollicis Tendon

Common disorders which respond well to Tendon Release Therapy™

- Tendinitis
- Hypertonicity (protective muscle spasm and spasticity)
- Muscular Dystrophies
- Hypotonias
- Fibromyalgias
- Tenosynovitis
- Tears and ruptures of tendons
- De Quervain–like syndromes
- Hallux Valgus–like syndromes
- Tendon Calcifications, such as calcification of the supraspinatus tendon and bicipital tendon calcification.

CHAPTER 26

MUSCLE RHYTHM THERAPY

About Circadian Rhythms

Every system in the human body has a circadian rhythm. The arterial pulse, the cranial rhythmic impulse, Myofascial Mapping™, visceral motility, brain and spinal cord motility are often assessed by manual practitioners. Frank Lowen (Biologic Analogs™) discovered the rhythm of muscles.

Lowen first described this rhythm in 1997 as a piston-like motility. When the muscle is palpated at the origin and musculotendinous insertion, there is a *cycle* which consists of: (a) *a shortening phase,* and (b) *an elongation phase.* This is possibly the cyclic motility of actin and myosin protein locking and unlocking which is required for muscle fiber contraction.

This rhythm, the piston-like shortening and elongation of the muscle, is not a reflection of a voluntary muscle contracting on demand, and relaxing upon demand. This motility, this cyclic motion, is a reflection of the normal status of tone in the muscle at all times. This rhythm will be present throughout a 24 hour day. This rhythm does not change during rest, sleep, movement.

This Muscle Rhythm™ will have a typical amplitude of shortening and elongation of approximately one third (1/3) the normal resting length of the muscle fiber. This means that during the shortening phase of the cycle, the muscle will decrease its length so that it shortens down to two thirds (2/3) of its normal resting length. When the muscle has been treated with Strain and Counterstrain and it is not in a state of muscle spasm, the Muscle Rhythm™ is healthier. When the Muscle Rhythm™ is a reflection of a more healthy muscle, the shortening phase of the cycle is enhanced, i.e. the muscle will be-

come two thirds (2/3) its length. When there is spasm of the muscle, the muscle will not shorten optimally during the shortening phase of the cycle. The muscle is this case might shorten only one sixth (1/6) or less. This means, when the muscle is in a state of protective muscle spasm, the amplitude of shortening and elongation varies from that of a healthy muscle not in a state of spasm.

This area of muscle function requires research in a laboratory setting. This Muscle Rhythm™ is a reflection of the health of the sarcomeres of that muscle. If there is hyperactivity of the myotatic reflex arc, the alpha or gamma neuron, the Muscle Rhythm™ will be compromised. If there is a protein disorder affecting the actin and myosin, the Muscle Rhythm™ will be compromised. If there is a supraspinal facilitation or inhibition problem, for example with CVA and spinal cord injury, the Muscle Rhythm™ will be compromised.

Treatment with Muscle Rhythm Therapy™

Treatment with Muscle Rhythm Therapy™ is simple, but requires good palpation skills. There are three planes that can be assessed and treated with Muscle Rhythm Therapy™. Each phase of the cycle is approximately 5–7 seconds, so that the duration of the cycle of the Muscle Rhythm™ is 10–14 seconds. There are approximately 6 cycles per minute. The first plane that can be palpated via this rhythm is the elongation and contraction of the muscle. The piston-like motion of the muscle on this plane can be palpated in a superior/inferior direction in relationship to the muscle. The second plane of the Muscle Rhythm™ is the widening and narrowing of the muscle. This plane can be palpated in a medial/lateral direction in relationship to the muscle. The third and last plane of the Muscle Rhythm™ can be palpated in an anterior/posterior direction in relationship to the muscle.

Variations of Muscle Rhythm™ affected by dysfunction:

1. When there is severe hypertonicity of the muscle, affected by hyperactivity on the myotatic reflex arc, the rhythm will have increased frequency.
2. When there is hypertonicity of the muscle, affected by supraspinal disinhibition, as with CVA, the rhythm will have increased frequency.
3. When there is no innervation of the muscle, as in paralysis secondary to peripheral neuron denervation, there will be no Muscle Rhythm.™
4. When there is spinal cord injury, with abnormal peripheral nerve innervation, the Muscle Rhythm™ will have decreased frequency.
5. When there is peripheral nerve fibrosis, the Muscle Rhythm™ will have decreased frequency.
6. When there is sarcomere dysfunction, the rhythm will have decreased frequency.
7. When there is any disorder affecting the Muscle Rhythm™, the amplitude of the shortening and elongation phases will be decreased.
8. When there is any disorder affecting the Muscle Rhythm™, the force of the rhythm is decreased.

Treatment is best performed as a an *indirect* technique. Each part of the muscle, the proximal and the distal portions, will be on a different vector of shortening and elongation. There are two methods for treating Muscle Rhythm™. One method is via *direct* method and utilizes *Induction* which was first developed by JeanPierre Barral. This method enhances the motion of each part of the Muscle Rhythm™ by augmenting the movement pattern of the proximal and of the distal parts of the muscle, individually, at the same time. The second method that utilizes *indirect* treatment of the Muscle Rhythm™ was developed by Sharon Weiselfish-Giammatteo. This approach is called *Resistence Therapy*™. Resistence Therapy™ is utilized by palpating the Muscle Rhythm™ and then performing a microsecond resistence to the rhythm anywhere in the cycle. The rhythm may respond in the following ways: 1. the Muscle Rhythm™ will be augmented immediately following the Resistence Therapy™, 2. the Muscle Rhythm™ will go into a self-corrective mode referred to as a *still point,* and will shut down temporarily to allow more internal changes to occur. After the still point ends and the rhythm turns back on, the result will be an augmentation of the Muscle Rhythm™.

CHAPTER 27

PROCEDURES AND PROTOCOLS
with Advanced Strain and Counterstrain Technique

The following Procedures and Protocols section is to be followed when there are physical motion limitations. Strain and Counterstrain Technique is performed for the purpose of increasing motion. In addition, there are now manners in which to re-educate active motion, and strengthen movement, with the use of the Synchronizers© presented in this book. It is now possible to utilize Strain/Counterstrain to improve active motion in cases of hypotonia, when there is no evidence of hypertonicity.

Dr. Lawrence Jones contributed an exceptional gift with Strain and Counterstrain Technique. Health care practitioners are able to facilitate normal movement for all persons who are suffering from pain and disability due to hypertonicity. This contribution is enormous. The resulting motion, increased functional capacity, decreased pain during movement, and tension reduction from de-facilitation are all the direct outcomes of this procedure. Dr. Jones added his insight from osteopathy, and correlated this technique with certain medical model symptoms, such as heartburn and indigestion and other symptoms.

Weiselfish-Giammatteo used this approach to treat postural deviations and deformities, achieving excellent results with scoliosis and other difficult postural dysfunctions. From this model of posture which responded to Strain and Counterstrain Technique, she developed a mechanical model called the Corrective Kinesiologic model for Strain and Counterstrain Technique. It is not necessary to use the painful tender points when working with this model. The understanding gained regarding the significant, profound effect on posture and motion due to hypertonicity was attained with this model.

Weiselfish-Giammatteo also developed a neurologic based model. The following recounts her first discovery in 1982 of the effect on severe neurologic phenomena with Strain and Counterstrain Technique. There is a common occurrence with the hemiplegic patient: they develop a subluxation of the hemiplegic shoulder. Bertha Bobath considered that a subluxed hemiplegic shoulder is the direct result of the hypertonicity of the latissimus dorsi muscle in a flaccid and low tone shoulder girdle. Because the latissimus dorsi is the only depressor of the humeral head, this is a reasonable hypothesis. Weiselfish-Giammatteo used the Strain and Counterstrain Technique for the latissimus dorsi on over a hundred hemiplegic shoulders during the years between 1982 and 1997. The positive results are astounding. The subluxation of the hemiplegic shoulder can be eliminated, not only reduced, with the Strain and Counterstrain approach. During the years, protocols were designed by Weiselfish-Giammatteo for utilization of this Technique with the neurologic, pediatric and geriatric patient population. For example, when use of Strain and Counterstrain occurs in "correct" kinesiologic sequence, there are better results, and there are minimal or no treatment reactions or discomfort. An example of "correct" kinesiologic sequence: When the protraction of the shoulder girdle is first eliminated with the second depressed rib technique (which affects the tone of the pectoralis minor), followed by the technique for the subscapularis in order to attain improved posterior position of the humeral head in the glenoid fossa, and after that treatment of the latissimus dorsi is performed, there is almost a 100% success rate in the reduction of the subluxation of the glenohumeral joint.

Weiselfish-Giammatteo continued her research with the neurologic patient population and discovered a Synergic Pattern Imprint™ (for further explanation, refer to Chapter 1) with all persons: orthopedic, neurologic, geriatric, chronic pain, sports medicine, pediatric and other. This pattern is the typical response of the human body as it responds to facilitation, which is due to excessive afferent discharge. This pattern is the same whether or not the cause of the afferent discharge abnormality is neuromusculoskeletalfascial dysfunction, or reduction of supraspinal inhibition. Hyperactivity of the myotatic reflex arc. The results are similar: the body takes on typical posture secondary to efferent gain (excessive alpha and gamma stimulation). When Strain and Counterstrain techniques are used on any patient population, there is a decrease in the presentation of this pattern, or an elimination of this pattern. The hypertonicity of spasticity can be successfully treated when the Synergic Pattern Imprint™ is 'released' with Strain and Counterstrain Technique.

Weiselfish-Giammatteo first observed Synchronizers™ in 1994. There are Synchronizers concealed in the body; they are reflexes which have major controlling influences over body functions. These Synchronizers™ are presented in Biologic Analogs courses, via Therapeutic Horizons. Weiselfish-Giammatteo has uncovered many Synchronizers™, two of which are significant in normalizing muscle function and are presented in this book. Weiselfish-Giammatteo hypothesizes that these two Synchronizers™ are responsible for: normalization of the actin and myosin locking and unlocking mechanism, and normalization of tetanic flow of impulses into the motor end plate. She hopes that future research by neuroscientists will further investigate these Synchronizers™ in controlled laboratory studies (for further explanation, refer to Chapter 2).

The following procedures and protocols are some of many which have been in development since 1984.

Anterior Compartment Syndrome

Anterior Compartment Syndrome is almost always a Double Crush Phenomenon. This phenomenon describes the proximal compression of the neural tissue which is causing the distal compromise of the neural mobility. In other words, because the brachial plexus is compressed at the thoracic inlet (between the anterior and middle scalenes; or within the costoclavicualr joint space; or underneath the pectoralis minor) the mobility of the distal median and ulnar nerves is decreased. Always treat anterior compartment syndrome with the Thoracic Outlet Protocol outlined in this text. If there is residual discomfort, or if the EMG and nerve conduction is not yet normal, add the following techniques to the protocol for Anterior Compartment Syndrome.

**Thoracic Outlet Protocol
(in Procedures and Protocols)**
plus
Jones Strain and Counterstrain Techniques
Long Head of the Biceps
Radial Head
Medial Epicondyle
Anterior Wrist Techniques
Advanced Strain/Counterstrain Techniques
Cervical and Upper extremity arteries, veins,
    lymph

INTEGRATIVE MANUAL THERAPY™

There is often compromised mobility of the peripheral nerves, especially the median nerve and the ulnar nerve, in Anterior Compartment Syndrome. Neural Tension Techniques (Elvey; Butler; Weiselfish-Giammatteo) will give extra-neural mobility. When there is intra-neural fibrosis of the median and/or ulnar nerves, the EMG and nerve conduction velocity tests will remain abnormal. The technique of choice to eliminate intra-neural fibrosis of the median and ulnar nerves is Neural Tension Techniques with Neurofascial Process™ (Weiselfish-Giammatteo). There may also be fascial dysfunction of the anterior compartment soft tissue. Myofascial Release, especially the 3-Planar Fascial Fulcrum Technique™ (Weiselfish-Giammatteo) can be utilized to normalize the flexibility of the connective tissue of the forearm. There may remain tension of the interosseous membrane. The Hanging Technique (Myofascial Release, Weiselfish-Giammatteo) will normalize the tension of the interosseous membrane.

Cardiac Syndromes

A cardiac syndrome includes all signs and symptoms due to pericardial and heart mobility and motility dysfunction. Tissue tension surrounding the heart will affect muscle, connective tissue, ligaments, and more. Signs are evident at the neck, thorax and rib cage, and left upper extremity. Assess right cervical rotation and right cervical side bending for limitations of motion. Assess cervical and thoracic spine extension, which will be limited when heart and pericardial tissue is tense. Right thoracic rotation and side bending, and left thoracic rotation and side bending will be limited. Rib cage excursion will be compromised on the left side. There will be limitations of all end ranges of motion of the left shoulder girdle. Often, pain or paresthesia will affect the left upper extremity function. There may be an apparent compromise of cardiopulmonary endurance, although this may not be evident. Recommendations from the developers of Advanced Strain/Counterstrain Technique, Giammatteo and Weiselfish-Giammatteo: assess mobility and motility of the tissues and structures of the cervical and thoracic spine, the rib cage, the left upper extremity. Institute the following protocol when there is compromised mobility and motility.

Phase One

Jones' Strain and Counterstrain Techniques
Anterior Thoracic techniques from Anterior First Thoracic through Anterior Sixth Thoracic
Anterior Cervical techniques
Descended Rib Techniques, especially left side
Elevated Rib Techniques, especially left side
Second Depressed Rib, left
Subscapularis, left
Latissimus Dorsi, left
Long Head of Biceps, left

When the major stresses and tensions have been released, continue to Phase Two: the Advanced Strain/Counterstrain Technique.

Phase Two

Advanced Strain/Counterstrain Technique
Pelvic Diaphragm, bilateral
Respiratory Abdominal Diaphragm, bilateral
Thoracic Inlet, bilateral
Cranial Diaphragm, bilateral
Heart 1
Subclavius, bilateral
Aorta
Inferior Vena Cava
Superior Vena Cava
Circulatory Vessels of the Chest Cavity
Circulatory Vessels of the Abdomen
Circulatory Vessels of the Neck
Chest Cavity Lymphatic Vessels
Abdomenal Lymphatic Vessels
Neck Lymphatic Vessels
Intraventricular Coronary Arteries
Left Coronary Arteries
Left Anterior Descending Coronary Artery
Marginal Coronary Arteries
Posterior Descending Coronary Arteries
Right Coronary Artery
Right Marginal Coronary Artery
Subclavian Arteries
Superior Veins of the Trunk
Inferior Alveolar Veins
Posterior Superior Alveolar Veins
Arteries of the lungs
Arteries of the Capsules of Kidneys
Renal Arteries
Portal Veins
Common Carotid Arteries
Iliac Arteries
Proximal Femoral Arteries
Arteries of the Arm

INTEGRATIVE MANUAL THERAPY™

The developers of Advanced Strain/Counterstrain Technique, Giammatteo and Weiselfish-Giammatteo, have utilized these techniques for several years with various clients in different patient populations. There have not been any side effects. When procedures are sequenced appropriately, there are not any treatment reactions.

The only significant precaution: treat the striatal muscles innervated by the voluntary nervous system before treating the smooth muscles of the arteries which are innervated by the autonomic nervous system. The body can have good ranges of spinal movement, and good ranges of motion of the extremity joints when treated with Jones Strain and Counterstrain Technique. *Restore joint mobility and ranges of motion of the spine and rib cage and extremities prior to therapeutic intervention with Advanced Strain/Counterstrain for the arteries and veins and lymph musculature.* The practitioner can proceed without concern when the client remains alert and can verbalize and articulate how well he/ she is feeling. If the practitioner is using these techniques with a patient who is not conscious, or verbal and articulate, monitor pulse and blood pressure. After each technique there should be status quo, or improved blood pressure as well as radial pulse. The practitioners who are not educated in the medical model of assessment, diagnosis and treatment of cardiac disorder and disease will be limited to evaluation of motion: joint mobility, soft tissue flexibility, ranges of motion, strength, endurance. Other practitioners can utilize varied approaches for assessment and pre and post testing.

Carpal Tunnel Syndrome

Carpal Tunnel Syndrome is almost always a Double Crush Phenomenon. This phenomenon describes the proximal compression of the neural tissue which is causing the distal compromise of the neural mobility. In other words, because the brachial plexus is compressed at the thoracic inlet (between the anterior and middle scalenes; or within the costoclavicular joint space; or underneath the pectoralis minor) the mobility of the distal median and ulnar nerves is decreased. Always treat carpal tunnel syndrome with the Thoracic Outlet Protocol outlined in this text. If there is residual discomfort, or if the EMG and nerve conduction is not yet normal, add the following techniques to the protocol for Carpal Tunnel Syndrome.

Thoracic Outlet Protocol
(in Procedures and Protocols)
plus
Jones' Strain and Counterstrain Techniques
Long Head of the Biceps
Radial Head
Medial Epicondyle
Anterior Wrist Techniques
Advanced Strain and Counterstrain Technique
Cervical and Upper Extremity arteries, veins,
    lymph

INTEGRATIVE MANUAL THERAPY™

There is often compromised mobility of the peripheral nerves, especially the median nerve and the ulnar nerve, in Carpal Tunnel Syndrome. Neural Tension Techniques (Elvey; Butler; Weiselfish-Giammatteo) will give extra-neural mobility. When there is intra-neural fibrosis of the median and/or ulnar nerves, the EMG and nerve conduction velocity tests will remain abnormal. The technique of choice to eliminate intra-neural fibrosis of the median and ulnar nerves is Neural Tension Techniques with Neurofascial Process™ (Weiselfish-Giammatteo). There may also be fascial dysfunction of the flexor retinaculum. Myofascial Release, especially the 3-Planar Fascial Fulcrum™ Technique (Weiselfish-Giammatteo) can be utilized to normalize the flexibility of the carpal retinaculum.

Headaches

Headaches ALWAYS have a component of sacral dysfunction. There is often compromise of *pelvic joint mobility* (pubic symphysis and right and left iliosacral joints). There is always compromise of *sacral joint mobility* (right and left sacroiliac joints; lumbosacral junction; sacrococcygeal joint). The most effective and efficient manner to *correct biomechanical dysfunction of the pelvic and sacral joints is MUSCLE ENERGY 'Beyond' TECHNIQUE*, which can be studied in DCR (Dialogues in Contemporary Rehabilitation courses), in the book *Manual Therapy for the Pelvis, Sacrum, Cervical, Thoracic and Lumbar Spine with Muscle Energy Technique* (Weiselfish-Giammatteo), or in the videos (4) covering Muscle Energy and 'Beyond' Technique (Weiselfish-Giammatteo). When the practitioner does not practice this approach, the manner to achieve mobility of the pelvic and sacral joints with Strain and Counterstrain Technique is as follows:

Phase One

Jones Strain and Counterstrain Technique
Iliacus
Anterior Fifth Lumbar
Medial Hamstrings
Adductors
Gluteus Medius
Piriformis
Posterior Sacral Techniques (PS1 right and left,
    PS2, PS3, PS4, PS5 right and left)

After these techniques are performed, perform *Disc Therapy*™ at the spinal junctions with Advanced Strain/Counterstrain Technique.

Phase Two

Advanced Strain/Counterstrain Technique
Disc Therapy™
L5
S1
T12
L1
C7
T1

Then perform all of the Strain and Counterstrain techniques for the *upper cervicals and cranium*, as follows:

Phase Three

Jones Strain and Counterstrain Technique
C1 (all Jones techniques)
Inion

Then continue with Advanced Strain/Counterstrain techniques.

Phase Four

Advanced Strain/Counterstrain Techniques
Pelvic Diaphragm
Respiratory Abdominal Diaphragm
Thoracic Inlet
Cranial Diaphragm
Tympanic Membrane
Anterior and Posterior Spinal Arteries
Circulatory Vessels of the Neck
Circulatory Vessels of the Cranial Vault

Migraine Headaches

Migraine headaches ALWAYS have a significant component of severe sacral dysfunction. There is often compromise of *pelvic joint mobility* (pubic symphysis and right and left iliosacral joints). There is always significant compromise of *sacral joint mobility* (right and left sacroiliac joints; lumbosacral junction; sacrococcygeal joint). The most effective and efficient manner to *correct biomechanical dysfunction of the pelvic and sacral joints is MUSCLE ENERGY and 'Beyond' TECHNIQUE* which can be studied in DCR (Dialogues in Contemporary Rehabilitation courses), in the book *Manual Therapy for the Pelvis, Sacrum, Cervical, Thoracic and Lumbar Spine with Muscle Energy Technique* (Weiselfish-Giammatteo), or in the videos (4) covering Muscle Energy and 'Beyond' Technique (Weiselfish-Giammatteo). When the practitioner does not practice this approach, the manner to achieve mobility of the pelvic and sacral joints with Strain and Counterstrain Technique is as follows:

Phase One

Jones' Strain and Counterstrain Technique
Iliacus
Anterior Fifth Lumbar
Medial Hamstrings
Adductors
Gluteus Medius
Piriformis
Posterior Sacral Techniques (PS1 right and left, PS2, PS3, PS4, PS5 right and left)

After these techniques are performed, perform *Disc Therapy*™ at the spinal junctions with Advanced Strain/Counterstrain Technique.

Phase Two

Advanced Strain/Counterstrain Technique
Disc Therapy™
L5

S1
T12
L1
C7
T1

Then perform all of the Strain and Counterstrain techniques for the *upper cervicals and cranium*, as follows:

Phase Three

Jones' Strain and Counterstrain Technique
C1 (all Jones techniques)
Inion
Occipitomastoid
Coronal
Lambda
Supraorbital
Infraorbital
Masseter
(All other appropriate Jones Strain and Counterstrain of the cranium and face.)

Then continue with Advanced Strain/Counterstrain techniques.

Phase Four

Advanced Strain/Counterstrain Techniques
Pelvic Diaphragm
Respiratory Abdominal Diaphragm
Thoracic Inlet
Subclavius
Subclavian Artery
Hilum of the Lungs
Cranial Diaphragm
Tympanic Membrane
Anterior and Posterior Spinal Arteries
Anterior and Posterio Spinal Veins
Sacral-Coccyx Artery
Accessory Meningeal Artery
Renal Artery
Circulatory Vessels of the Neck
Circulatory Vessels of the Cranial Vault
Circulatory Vessels of the Facial Vault

Superficial Cerebral Veins
Superficial Veins of the Head
Neck Lymphatic Vessels
Cranium and Intra-cranial Lymphatic Vessels
Heart 1
Aorta
Inferior Vena Cava
Superior Vena Cava
Ocular Muscles (Eye 1, Eye 2, Eye 3, Eye 4)
Common Carotid Artery
External Carotid Artery
Internal Carotid Artery
Arteries of the Brain
Artery of Circle of Willis
Basilar Artery
Arteries of the Eye

INTEGRATIVE MANUAL THERAPY™

The significance of biomechanical dysfunction of the sacrum cannot be overstated. Please correct the joint dysfunction of the sacroiliac joints and the lumbosacral junction in all patients with head signs and symptoms. They have found that the most effective and efficient manner in which to restore biomechanical integrity of the pelvis and sacrum is Muscle Energy and 'Beyond' Technique. This process can be learned in various ways: (1) Manual Therapy for the Pelvis, Sacrum, Cervical, Thoracic and Lumbar Spine with Muscle Energy Technique, Weiselfish-Giammatteo; (2) Courses with Dialogues in Contemporary Rehabilitation (DCR); (3) Videos on Muscle Energy and 'Beyond' Technique, Weiselfish-Giammatteo, with Northeast Seminars. When biomechanics have been optimally restored, Jones Strain and Counterstrain Technique is good for increasing joint mobility of all spinal joints.

Reflex Sympathetic Dystrophy

Phase One

Jones' Strain and Counterstrain Techniques
Anterior First Thoracic
Anterior Cervicals: Anterior Fourth through eighth
Lateral Cervicals: all
Elevated First Rib
Anterior Acromioclavicular
Posterior Acromioclavicular
Second Depressed Rib (Pectoralis Minor)
Subscapularis
Latissimus Dorsi
Posterior First Thoracic
Inion

INTEGRATIVE MANUAL THERAPY™

The Brachial Plexus can be compressed in certain typical regions which will contribute to the pain and paresthesia of the arm in Thoracic Outlet Syndrome, which is always part of Reflex Sympathetic Dystrophy. Spinal cord fibrosis is a component of the compromise, contributing to the mechanical neural tension. Spinal cord fibrosis is addressed with cranial therapy. An excellent technique is Neurofascial Release Sagittal Plane™ (Weiselfish-Giammatteo). Another approach can be learned in the Biologic Analog™ courses (Lowen, Weiselfish-Giammatteo). Some of the cervical spinal nerve roots are always compressed within the intervertebral neural foramina in Reflex Sympathetic Dystrophy, contributing to the signs and symptoms of Thoracic Outlet Syndrome. Nerve root impingements can be alleviated with Craniosacral Therapy (Upledger); with techniques from Biologic Analogs™; and with Strain and Counterstrain Technique. The Lateral Cervical Strain and Counterstrain techniques will eliminate the hypertonicity of the middle scalene musculature. This will open the intervertebral neural foramina. There are four (4) other typical anatomic sites of compression of the brachial plexus. The first site is between the middle and anterior scalenes. To eliminate the protective muscle spasm of the middle scalenes, perform the Lateral Cervical techniques. In order to eliminate the hypertonicity of the anterior scalenes, perform the Anterior Cervical techniques from Anterior Fourth Cervical through Anterior Eighth Cervical. The second site of compression of the brachial plexus is within the costo-clavicular joint space. The costoclavicular joint space is opened with the following Strain and Counterstrain techniques: Anterior First Thoracic; Anterior Sixth and Anterior Seventh techniques; Anterior Acromioclavicular Joint and Posterior Acromioclavicular Joint techniques; Lateral Cervical techniques. The next anatomic site of compression of the brachial plexus is underneath the pectoralis minor, which can be treated with the Second Depressed Rib technique. (Often this technique must be preceded with the Subscapularis technique). The last site of anatomic compression is in axilla, by a caudal displacement of the humeral head. This compression can be alleviated with the Latissimus Dorsi technique. The sympathetic ganglia anterior to the first costovertebral joint is always compromised in Reflex Sympathetic Dystrophy. The Posterior First Thoracic technique will affect this compression on the superior, middle and inferior ganglia. Hold the position for a De-Facilitated Fascial Release. The Inion technique will decompress the craniocervical junction, and a decompression of the brain stem will result, so that there will be an increase of parasympathetic tone.

Phase Two

Reflex Sympathetic Dystrophy is an advanced stage of Thoracic Outlet Syndrome, which is the complex problems which result due to compression of the brachial plexus. Often there is compromise of the vascular tissues as well as the neural tissue. With Reflex Sympathetic Dystrophy there is always compromise of the peripheral neural tissue, the arterial musculature, the muscles of the veins, and the lymphatic muscles. Neural Tension Techniques (Elvey; Butler; Weiselfish-Giammatteo) may be required to alleviate all of the extra-neural impingements and intra-neural fibrosis which is typically present with Reflex Sympathetic Dystrophy. Advanced Strain/Counterstrain Technique can be utilized in order to completely decompress the neurovascular tissues.

Advanced Strain/Counterstrain Techniques
Subclavius
Subclavian Artery
Pelvic Diaphragm

Respiratory Abdominal Diaphragm
Thoracic Inlet
Cranial Diaphragm
Chest Cavity Lymphatic Vessels
Artery of the Lung
Heart 1
Aorta
Inferior Vena Cava
Superior Vena Cava
Anterior and Posterior Spinal Arteries
Circulatory Vessels of the Neck
Circulatory Vessels of the Upper Extremity
Common Carotid Artery
External Carotid Artery
Internal Carotid Artery
Superficial Veins of the Neck
Superficial Veins of the Arm
Neck Lymphatic Vessels
Upper Extremity Lymphatic Vessels
Arteries of the Arm
Axillary Artery
Brachial Artery
Artery of Circle of Willis
Posterior Cerebral Artery
Disc Therapy™ for all the cervical and thoracic discs, especially low cervical, high thoracic.

INTEGRATIVE MANUAL THERAPY™

The elimination of hypertonicity of the subclavius muscle will decompress the subclavian artery which lies beneath the subclavius. The four diaphragms (pelvic, respiratory abdominal, thoracic inlet and cranial diaphragm) function together as a unit. When one diaphragm is in a state of hypertonicity, all of the diaphragms will be in a reflexive hypertonic state. Therefore, all of the diaphragms must be treated, bilateral, in order to completely alleviate the tension of the thoracic inlet. There is always hypertonicity of the musculature of the arteries and lymph vessels.

Respiratory Syndromes

A respiratory syndrome includes all signs and symptoms due to pulmonary, pleura and rib cage mobility and motility dysfunction. Tissue tension surrounding the lungs and pleura will affect muscle, connective tissue, ligaments, and more. Signs are evident at the neck, thorax and rib cage, right and left upper extremity. Assess bilateral cervical rotation and side bending for limitations of motion. Assess cervical and thoracic spine extension, which will be limited when lung and pleural tissue is tense. Bilateral thoracic rotation and side bending will be limited. Rib cage excursion will be compromised on both sides. There will be limitations of all end ranges of motion of the shoulder girdles. Often pain/or paresthesia will affect upper extremity function. There may be an apparent compromise of respiratory endurance, although this may not be evident. Recommendations from the developers of Advanced Strain/Counterstrain Technique, Giammatteo and Weiselfish-Giammatteo: assess mobility and motility of the tissues and structures of the cervical and thoracic spine, the rib cage, the upper extremities. Assess respiration. Institute the following protocol when there is compromised mobility and motility.

Phase One

Jones' Strain and Counterstrain Techniques
Anterior Thoracic techniques from Anterior
   First Thoracic through Anterior Sixth
   Thoracic
Anterior Cervical techniques
Descended Rib Techniques, especially left side
Elevated Rib Techniques, especially left side
Second Depressed Rib
Subscapularis
Latissimus Dorsi

When the major stresses and tensions have been released, continue with the Advanced Strain/Counterstrain Techniques.

Phase Two

Advanced Strain/Counterstrain Technique
Pelvic Diaphragm, bilateral
Respiratory Abdominal Diaphragm, bilateral
Thoracic Inlet, bilateral
Cranial Diaphragm, bilateral
Tympanic Membranes
Heart 1
Lung 1
Hilum of the Lung
Subclavius, bilateral
Aorta
Inferior Vena Cava
Superior Vena Cava
Subclavian Arteries
Circulatory Vessels of the Chest Cavity
Circulatory Vessels of the Abdomen
Circulatory Vessels of the Neck
Chest Cavity Lymphatic Vessels
Abdomenal Lymphatic Vessels
Neck Lymphatic Vessels
Superior Veins of the Trunk
Arteries of the lungs
Inferior Alveolar Veins
Posterior Superior Alveolar Veins
Common Carotid Arteries

INTEGRATIVE MANUAL THERAPY™

The developers of Advanced Strain/Counterstrain Technique, Giammatteo and Weiselfish-Giammatteo, have utilized these techniques for several years with various clients in different patient populations. There have not been any side effects. When procedures are sequenced appropriately, there are not any treatment reactions. *The only significant precaution: treat the striatal muscles innervated by the voluntary nervous system before treating the smooth muscles of the arteries which are innervated by the autonomic nervous system.* The body can have good ranges of spinal movement, and good ranges of motion of the extremity joints when treated with Jones Strain and Counterstrain Technique. *Restore joint mobility and ranges of motion of the spine and rib cage and extremities prior to therapeutic intervention with Advanced Strain/Counterstrain for the arteries and veins and lymph musculature.* The practitioner can proceed without concern when the client remains alert and can verbalize and articulate how well he/she is feeling. If the practitioner is using these techniques with a patient who is not conscious, or verbal and articulate, monitor pulse and blood pressure. After each technique there should be status quo, or improved blood pressure as well as radial pulse. The practitioners who are not educated in the medical model of assessment, diagnosis and treatment of cardiac disorder and disease will be limited to evaluation of motion: joint mobility, soft tissue flexibility, ranges of motion, strength, endurance. Other practitioners can utilize varied approaches for assessment and pre and post testing.

Spinal Syndromes

The developers of Advanced Strain/Counterstrain, Giammatteo and Weiselfish-Giammatteo, are convinced that correction of biomechanics of the pelvic joints (the pubic symphysis and the right and left iliosacral joints) and the sacral joints (the right and left sacroiliac joints, the lumbosacral junction, and the sacrococcygeal joint) should be treated prior to other intervention. They have found that the most effective and efficient manner in which to restore biomechanical integrity of the pelvis and sacrum is Muscle Energy and 'Beyond' Technique. This process can be learned in various ways: 1. Manual Therapy for the Pelvis, Sacrum, Cervical, Thoracic and Lumbar Spine with Muscle Energy Technique, Weiselfish-Giammatteo; 2. Courses with Dialogues in Contemporary Rehabilitation (DCR); 3. Videos on Muscle Energy and 'Beyond' Technique, Weiselfish-Giammatteo, with Northeast Seminars. When biomechanics has been optimally restored, Jones Strain and Counterstrain Technique is good for increasing joint mobility of all spinal joints. The following sequence can be followed.

Phase One

Jones' Strain and Counterstrain Techniques
Pelvis:
Iliacus
Medial Hamstrings
Adductors
Gluteus Medius
Sacrum:
Piriformis
Posterior Sacral Techniques (PS1 right and left, PS2, PS3, PS4, PS5 right and left)
Lumbar Spine:
Anterior Fifth Lumbar
Anterior and Posterior Lumbars
Latissimus Dorsi
Thoracic Spine:
Anterior and Posterior Thoracics
Anterior Twelfth Thoracic (Quadratus Lumborum)

Elevated Ribs
Descended Ribs
Cervical Spine:
Anterior and Posterior Cervicals
Lateral Cervicals

Phase Two

Advanced Strain/Counterstrain Technique
Pelvic Diaphragm
Respiratory Abdominal Diaphragm
Thoracic Inlet
Cranial Diaphragm
Disc Therapy: Phase One: for the Annulus
    Fibrosis of all Spinal Segments
Disc Therapy: Phase Two: for the Lining of the
    Disc of all Spinal Segments
Anterior and Posterior Spinal Arteries
Anterior and Posterior Spinal Veins
Sacro-Coccyx Artery (Middle Sacral Artery)
Middle Meningeal Artery
Accessory Meningeal Artery (Pial Arterial
    Plexus)

INTEGRATIVE MANUAL THERAPY™

Spinal Syndromes can include low back pain with or without sciatica, thoracic pain, cervical syndrome and neck pain, tension headaches; spinal cord problems including quadriplegia and quadriparesis, paraplegia and paraparesis, and degenerative diseases such as Multiple Sclerosis. Besides intervention with Muscle Energy and 'Beyond' Technique and Strain and Counterstrain Technique, and Advanced Strain/Counterstrain Technique, fascial release is an excellent adjunct. There is a spinal protocol which is presented in the DCR Myofascial Release Technique course which addresses the iliosacral joints, the sacrum, L5/S1, the thoracolumbar junction, the cervicothoracic junction, and the craniocervical junction. There are also Advanced Neural Tension Techniques (Weiselfish-Giammatteo) which address the neural tension of the plexii of the cervical, thoracic, lumbar and sacral regions. Giammatteo and Weiselfish-Giammatteo observed an extra-ordinary phenomenon, which reflects how the body protects vascular tissue. Evidence of spinal cord fibrosis may totally disappear when the spinal arteries and veins are treated with Advanced Strain/Counterstrain Technique. The neural tension was present because of arterial/venous compromise, and the spinal cord/ column was required to be in a state of contraction in order to alleviate tension on the spinal arteries and veins.

Speech and Swallowing Disorders

Dysphagia may be secondary to any type of neuromusculoskeletal dysfunction. Strain and Counterstrain Technique often has a remarkable effect on speech and swallowing, including: drooling, articulation and enunciation, tongue thrust, lisp, and more. The following sequence of techniques may facilitate changes for the practitioner.

Phase One

Jones' Strain and Counterstrain Technique
Anterior Cervical: Anterior Cervical One
     through Anterior Cervical Seven (All)
Inion
Coronal
Occipitomastoid
Lambda

Phase Two

Advanced Strain/Counterstrain Technique
Pelvic Diaphragm
Respiratory Abdomenal Diaphragm
Thoracic Inlet
Cranial Diaphragm
Subclavius
Myelohyoid
Elevation of the Thyroid Cartilage
Vocal Cords
Arytenoid Tendency to Adduct
Circulatory Vessels of the Neck
Circulatory Vessels of the Cranium
Circulatory Vessels of the Facial Vault

INTEGRATIVE MANUAL THERAPY™

Structural Rehabilitation to improve the potential for speech and swallowing must include the assessment of the following: (1) cranial and neuronal mobility and motility of the parietals, especially left (Broca's speech area); (2) cranial and neuronal mobility and motility of the brain stem; neural tension of the following cranial nerves: glossopharyngeal (#9), vagus (#10), hypoglossal (#12); (3)mobility of the hyoid bone, thyroid cartilage; (4) fascial dysfunction of the hyoid system.

Thoracic Outlet Syndrome

Phase One

Jones' Strain and Counterstrain Techniques
Anterior First Thoracic
Anterior Cervicals: Anterior Fourth through
     eighth
Lateral Cervicals: all
Elevated First Rib
Anterior Acromioclavicular
Posterior Acromioclavicular
Second Depressed Rib (Pectoralis Minor)
Subscapularis
Latissimus Dorsi

INTEGRATIVE MANUAL THERAPY™

The Brachial Plexus can be compressed in certain typical regions which will contribute to the pain and paresthesia of the arm in Thoracic Outlet Syndrome. Often, spinal cord fibrosis is a component of the compromise, contributing to the mechanical neural tension. Spinal cord fibrosis is addressed with cranial therapy. An excellent technique is Neurofascial Release Sagittal Plane™ (Weiselfish-Giammatteo). Also, the spinal nerve roots can be compressed within the intervertebral neural foramina contributing to the signs and symptoms of Thoracic Outlet Syndrome. Nerve root impingements can be alleviated with Craniosacral Therapy (Upledger); with techniques from Biologic Analogs™; and with Strain and Counterstrain Technique. The Lateral Cervical Strain and Counterstrain techniques will eliminate the hypertonicity of the middle scalene musculature. This will open the intervertebral neural foramina. There are four (4) other typical anatomic sites of compression of the brachial plexus. The first site is between the middle and anterior scalenes. To eliminate the protective muscle spasm of the middle scalenes, perform the Lateral Cervical techniques. In order to eliminate the hypertonicity of the anterior scalenes, perform the Anterior Cervical techniques from Anterior Fourth Cervical through Anterior Eighth Cervical. The second site of compression of the brachial plexus is within the costoclavicular joint space. The costoclavicular joint space is opened with the following Strain and Counterstrain techniques: Anterior First Thoracic; Anterior Sixth and Anterior Seventh techniques; Anterior Acromioclavicular Joint and Posterior Acromioclavicular Joint techniques;

Lateral Cervical techniques. The next anatomic site of compression of the brachial plexus is underneath the pectoralis minor, which can be treated with the Second Depressed Rib technique. (Often this technique must be preceded with the Subscapularis technique). The last site of anatomic compression is in axilla, by a caudal displacement of the humeral head. This compression can be alleviated with the Latissimus Dorsi technique.

Phase Two

Thoracic Outlet Syndrome is the complex problems which result due to compression of the brachial plexus. Often there is compromise of the vascular tissues as well as the neural tissue. Advanced Strain/Counterstrain Technique can be utilized in order to completely decompress the neurovascular tissues.

Advanced Strain/Counterstrain Techniques
Subclavius
Subclavian Artery
Pelvic Diaphragm
Respiratory Abdominal Diaphragm
Thoracic Inlet
Cranial Diaphragm
Circulatory Vessels of the Neck
Circulatory Vessels of the Upper Extremity
Common Carotid Artery
External Carotid Artery
Internal Carotid Artery
Superficial Veins of the Neck
Superficial Veins of the Arm
Neck Lymphatic Vessels
Upper Extremity Lymphatic Vessels
Disc Therapy™ for the cervical and lower
    thoracic discs

INTEGRATIVE MANUAL THERAPY™

The elimination of hypertonicity of the subclavius muscle will decompress the subclavian artery which lies beneath the subclavius. The four diaphragms (pelvic, respiratory abdominal, thoracic inlet, and cranial diaphragm) function together as a unit. When one diaphragm is in a state of hypertonicity, all of the diaphragms will be in a reflexive hypertonic state.

Therefore, all of the diaphragms must be treated, bilateral, in order to completely alleviate the tension of the thoracic inlet.

Vision Disorders

Often visual disorders are secondary to structural dysfunction which can be addressed by manual practitioners. The following protocol has been found helpful by the developers of Advanced Strain/Counterstrain Technique.

Phase One

Jones' Strain and Counterstrain Technique
Coronal
Supra-orbital
Infra-orbital

Phase Two

Advanced Strain/Counterstrain Technique
Pelvic Diaphragm
Respiratory Abdominal Diaphragm
Thoracic Inlet
Cranial Diaphragm
Eye 1
Eye 2
Eye 3
Eye 4
Aorta
Subclavius
Subclavian Artery
Common Carotid Artery
Internal Carotid Artery
Circle of Willis
Basilar Artery
Anterior Cerebral Artery
Circulatory Vessels of the Neck
Circulatory Vessels of the Cranial Vault
Circulatory Vessels of the Facial Vault
Cranium and Intra-Cranial Lymphatic Vessels
Facial Lymphatic Vessels
Neck Lymphatic Vessels
Superficial Veins of the Head
Superficial Veins of the Face
Arteries of the Eye
Ciliary Muscles
Lens of the Eye
Renal Artery

INTEGRATIVE MANUAL THERAPY™

The developers of Advanced Strain/Counterstrain Technique, Giammatteo and Weiselfish-Giammatteo, highly recommend intensive functional rehabilitation for vision therapy, including: (1) Behavioral optometry (neuro-optometry); (2) Meir Schneider's Self Healing approach for vision therapy.

INDEX

DIALOGUES IN CONTEMPORARY REHABILITATION

History of Dialogues in Contemporary Rehabilitation

DCR is the company for Integrative Manual Therapy™, the Integrated Systems Approach™, Integrative Diagnostics™, and 'Functional and Structural Rehabilitation'. Founded in the early 1980's by Mary Fiorentino, O.T.,R. Sharon Weiselfish-Giammatteo initiated a transformation in the educational process incorporated by DCR in 1986, when she received ownership from Mary. Faculty of DCR are trained in all areas of manual therapy, experts in the fields of orthopedics and sports medicine, chronic pain, neuro-rehabilitation, pediatrics, geriatrics, women's and men's health issues, cardiopulmonary rehabilitation and more. Almost 100% of the material offered by DCR has been developed, research and present-day-results performed, at Regional Physical Therapy in Connecticut.

DCR Mission Statement

DCR offers hope, practice and purpose. Our goal is recovery; our intention is learning, teaching, and understanding. Our field of accomplishment is extended to client, family, community and world. We accept tomorrow's knowledge as today's quest. We are not hindered by greed, inhibitions, or belief systems. We are multi-denominational, cross-cultural, and non-racial in orientation. We wish to facilitate recovery from dysfunction through growth and development.

DCR Seminars

Biomechanics with: Muscle Energy and 'Beyond' Technique

MET1: Pelvis, Sacrum and Spine

MET2: Upper and Lower Extremities and Rib Cage

MET3: Advanced Biomechanics: Sacrum and Spine

MET4: Type III Biomechanical Dysfunction Spine and Extremities

Muscle and Circulation with Strain and Counterstrain Technique

SCS1: Strain and Counterstrain for Orthopedics and Neurologic Patient

SCS2: Advanced Strain/Counterstrain for Autonomic Nervous System

Connective Tissue with Myofascial Release, The 3-Planar Fascial Fulcrum™ Technique

MFR1: Myofascial Release for Orthopedic, Neurologic, Geriatric Patient

MFR2: Myofascial Mapping™ for Integrative Diagnostics™

Peripheral Nerve Tissue Tension: Hypomobility and Fibrosis

NTT2: Neural Tissue Tension Technique

Cranial and the Craniosacral System with: The Cranial Therapy Series

CTS1: Osseous, Suture, Joint ad Membrane

CTS2: Membrane, Fluid, Facial Valut and Cranial Gear-Complex

CTS3: Cranial Diaphragm Compression Syndromes; CSF Fluid: Production, Distribution and Absorption; Immunology

CTS4: Neuronal Regeneration, Cranial Nerves, and Neurotransmission

Organs with Visceral Mobilization

VMET1: Visceral Mobilization with Muscle Energy and 'Beyond'—Focus GI Tract

VMET2: Women's and Men's Health Issues

VMET3: Respiratory Rehabilitation

Compression Syndromes

COMP1: Compression Syndromes of the Upper Extremities

COMP2: Compression Syndromes of the Lower Extremities

COMP3: Diaphragm Compression Syndromes

NeuroRehabilitation

DMT: Developmental Manual Therapy for the Neurologic Patient

Integrative Diagnostics™

IDS: Integrative Diagnostic™ Series: Mapping™, Neurofascial Process™, Rx Plans

IDAP: Integrative Diagnostics™ for Applied Psychosynthesis

IDLB: Integrative Diagnostics™ for Lower Back

Integrative Seminars

IMTS: Integrative Manual Therapy™ for Neck, Thoracic Outlet, Shoulder and Upper Extremity

IMTUE/LESM: Integrative Manual Therapy™ for Upper and Lower Extremities in Sports Medicine

IMTCCC: Integrative Manual Therapy™ for Craniocervical, Craniofacial, Craniomandibular

NES & DCR Offer Adjunct Educational Material in Integrative Manual Therapy™

Books

Manual Therapy for the Pelvis, Sacrum, Cervical, Thoracic and Lumbar Spine, with Muscle Energy Technique—A Contemporary Clinical Analysis of Biomechanics by Sharon Weiselfish, Ph.D., P.T.

Integrative Manual Therapy™ for the Autonomic Nervous System and Related Disorders by Thomas Giammatteo, D.C. P.T., and Sharon Weiselfish-Giammatteo, Ph.D., P.T.

Integrative Manual Therapy™ for the Upper and Lower Extremities, Introducing Synergic Pattern Release™ with Strain and Counterstrain Technique and Muscle Energy and 'Beyond' Technique for the Peripheral Joints by Sharon Weiselfish-Giammatteo, Ph.D., P.T., edited by Thomas Giammatteo, D.C., P.T.

Videos

By Sharon Weiselfish-Giammatteo, Ph.D., P.T. Produced by Northeast Seminars

Muscle Energy Technique Series

#1 Pelvis

#2 Sacrum

#3 Thoracic and Lumbar Spine

#4 Cervical and Thoracic Spine

#5 Strain and Counterstrain for the Orthopedic and Neurologic Patient

#6 Myofascial Release, The 3-Planar Fascial Fulcrum™ Approach, for the Orthopedic, Neurologic and Geriatric Patient.

#7 Advanced Manual Therapy for the Low Back

#8 Integrative Manual Therapy™

#9 Manual Therapy for the Low Back: Standards for the Health Care Industry for the 21st Century

#10 Muscle Energy and 'Beyond' Technique for the Upper Extremities

#11 Muscle Energy and 'Beyond' Technique for the Lower Extremities

For further information regarding educational
products, please contact Northeast Seminars at:

Northeast Seminars
P.O. Box 522
East Hampstead, NH 03826
Tel: 800-272-2044
Fax: 603-329-7045
E-mail: neseminar@aol.com
Website: www.neseminars.com

For further information regarding DCR
seminars, please contact DCR at:

DCR
Dialogues in Contemporary Rehabilitation
800 Cottage Grove Rd
Bloomfield, CT 06002
Tel: 860-243-5220 / Fax: 860-243-5304
E-mail: dcrhealth@aol.com
Website: www.dcrhealth.com